Advance praise for *Caregiver'*

"Even for someone as supremely accomplished as scientist, inventor, and waterman Dr. Rob Yonover, nineteen years devoted to caring for his wife's MS seemed at the outset an outsized challenge. Where do you start? How do you endure? How do you create the best life for the one you love and will eventually lose, as they can no longer live the life the two of you had planned? *Caregiver's Survival Guide* is the hard-won, easy and entertaining to read, step-by-step how-to/ memoir of the Yonovers' intimate journey, wrapped up in a love letter to his late wife, Cindy. It's packed with practical advice and deep personal insights—all designed to provide focus and equilibrium in the face of the overwhelming. This is what you have to know as a caregiver to care not only for your loved one, but to also care for yourself."

—David Rensin, co-author of American hero Louis Zamperini's best-selling autobiography *Devil at My Heels*, and *All for a Few Perfect Waves*

"Based on research and nineteen years of experience, this family caregiving narrative provides an honest, compassionate, and humor-filled guide that will appeal to those involved in any kind of long-term care partnering. From how to source expert help and services, deal with extended family and visitors, to self-care, carving out a niche for joy, and managing grief, the *Caregiver's Survival Guide* illustrates how love, in very tricky times, can both sustain and enhance relationships."

—Cathie Borrie, author of *The Long Hello*

"An informative gem that can only inspire admiration for Dr. Rob Yonover's decades of full-time work keeping a loved one alive and a family together. Hard-won practical tips included."

—Ethan Podet, MD

"Caregiving is hard work under any circumstance, particularly so when the recipient is in a condition which declines. Just when you think you've reached your limit, caretaking demands increase. Beyond the incredible personal story of Rob Yonover's unexpected challenge, caretaking of his wife with MS, and raising his two young children, is the psychological process of finding one's resilient core. His story is a guide to all about redefining one's identity and values in an authentically sustainable way with everything at stake. Sustainable, because often the person saving another gets drowned themselves. I recommend the book as a highly readable, informative guide, a story of love and personal struggle filled with support, practical day-by-day tips, but most importantly a path to discovering one's own core resiliency."

—Wayne Giancaterino, PhD, clinical psychologist

"Caregiving is one of life's most brutal, yet fulfilling experiences. This honest, unflinching, yet humorous guide is sure to help others who are about to start their own journeys."

—Noriko Wada, active caregiver

"Rob's wry sense of humor, combined with his unflinching observations, are a refreshing departure from the usual literature. As a fellow caregiver, it's reassuring to see there are universal truths—I just wish I had this guide before starting on my own journey!"

—W. N., caregiver for parents suffering from dementia

Caregiver's Survival Guide

Caring for Yourself While Caring for a Loved One

ROBERT YONOVER, PhD, and ELLIE CROWE

Illustrations by Janet King
Foreword by Carlyn A. Tamura, PsyD

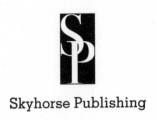

Skyhorse Publishing

Skyhorse Publishing books may be purchased in bulk at special discounts for sales promotion, corporate gifts, fund-raising, or educational purposes. Special editions can also be created to specifications. For details, contact the Special Sales Department, Skyhorse Publishing, 307 West 36th Street, 11th Floor, New York, NY 10018 or info@skyhorsepublishing.com.

Skyhorse® and Skyhorse Publishing® are registered trademarks of Skyhorse Publishing, Inc.®, a Delaware corporation.

Visit our website at www.skyhorsepublishing.com.

10 9 8 7 6 5 4 3 2 1

Library of Congress Cataloging-in-Publication Data

Names: Yonover, Robert, author. | Crowe, Ellie, author.
Title: Caregiver's survival guide: caring for yourself while caring for a loved one / Robert Yonover, PhD, and Ellie Crowe ; illustrations by Janet King; foreword by Carlyn A. Tamura, PsyD ; introduction by Robert Yonover, PhD.
Description: New York: Skyhorse Publishing, [2018] | Includes bibliographical references.
Identifiers: LCCN 2018005562| ISBN 9781510731776 (pbk.: alk. paper) | ISBN 9781510731783 (ebook)
Subjects: LCSH: Caregivers--Hawaii—Popular works. | Male caregivers—Hawaii--Popular works. | Caregivers—Family relationships—Popular works.
Classification: LCC HV1441.8.U5 Y66 2018 | DDC 649.8—dc23 LC record available at https://lccn.loc.gov/2018005562

Cover design by Mona Lin

Print ISBN: 978-1-5107-3177-6
Ebook ISBN: 978-1-5107-3178-3

Printed in the United States of America

*To Our Son and Daughter
and to All the Children of Parents with Medical Challenges*
—Rob Yonover

Contents

Foreword   xi

Introduction   xiii

SECTION 1—TWO IN DEEP   1

Chapter 1—Hold On to the Foundations of
Your Relationship   3
  Happy, Loving Couple   3

Chapter 2—Dealing with Heavy News   7
  Brain Stem Lesion   7
  Telling Your Family and Friends   7
  Short-Term vs. Long-Term Conditions   9

Chapter 3—Dealing with Daily Challenges   13
  Loss of Mobility and the Dreaded Wheelchair   13
  Developing My Feminine Side   15

Chapter 4—Why Me? And the Blame Game   17

Chapter 5—Take Stock of Your Ship   21
  How's Your Ship?   22
  Assess the Mental Health of Your Team   24

Children's Needs   25
Assess Your Own Health   26
Manage Caregiver Stress   28

Chapter 6—Caregiver Mental Health Breaks   **31**
Caregiver Escapes   32
Escape into Nature   34
Go to Your Village   35

Chapter 7—Counseling   **39**
Taking Care of Yourself   40
Value What You Provide   40

Chapter 8—Take Stock of Your Finances   **43**
Finances—Or the Money Pit   43
Use Your Caregiving Dollars Wisely   44
Pick Your Priorities   45
Seek Professional Advice   46

Chapter 9—Seek Ways to Adapt and Still Enjoy Life **47**
Carve Your Joy Niche   49
Keep It Light   49
Entertainment   50
Exercise   52
Cycling System   53
Help Care Recipient Keep a Favorite Activity   54
Travel Strategies and Fabio   56

Chapter 10—Mental Health and Staying Sane   **59**
Ignore and Distract   61
Staying Sane   62

Chapter 11—The Social Aspect   **65**
Visitors: The Good, the Bad, and the Clueless   66
Kindred Spirit—Louie Zamperini   67

Chapter 12—Chasing Rainbows   69
   Dead Man Surfing   69
   Israeli Dream   71
   Quacks 'R' Us   73

Chapter 13—Frustration and Loss   75
   Six-Day War, 2012   76
   Bub and Lovie Sitcom, 2015   77

SECTION 2—BASIC TASKS   81

Chapter 14—Gut Check and the Daily Challenge   83
   Trust Your Instincts   84
   Feeding   85
   Sleeping   86
   Bathroom and Beyond   89
   Public Bathrooms   92
   Bathing   93
   Transfers   96

Chapter 15—Medications and Marijuana   99
   Avoid Problems with Pills   100

SECTION 3—REACH OUT FOR HELP   103

Chapter 16—Seek Expert Help and Advice   105
   Seek Financial Advice   105
   Seek Legal Advice   106
   Public Benefits   106
     Services for Veterans 106
     Community Services   107
     Adult Day Care   108
     Medicare In-Home Part-Time Nursing or
       Rehabilitative Care   109

Community Care Services 110
Hospice and Medicare 110
Family and Medical Leave Act 111
Insurance 111
Free or Discounted Services for Seniors or Caregivers 112

Chapter 17—Nurses and Helpers 117
Live-In Help at Care Recipient's Home 117
Suggestions for Employing Live-In Help 117
Considering Applicants 118
Interview 118
Checking References 119
Physical Help at Home 120
Hiring Help 120
Privacy 121
Help from Family 122

Chapter 18—Doctors 125
Dealing with Doctors 127
Choosing a Doctor 128
Doctor's Visits 129

Chapter 19—Fight for Your Rights and Causes 131

SECTION 4—GRIEVE AND THEN CREATE NEW DREAMS **133**

Chapter 20—Love, Loss, and Lessons Learned 135

Chapter 21—Caregiving, A Daughter's Perspective, Kera Yonover 137

Index 141

Foreword

BY CARLYN A. TAMURA, PsyD
Clinical Psychologist, Child and Family Therapist

If you are a caregiver of a spouse, parent, or child with a serious illness, don't think twice before you read this book. In *Caregiver's Survival Guide*, Robert Yonover, PhD, presents a humanistic, compassionate, and practical look at the tools one needs to survive and thrive on the emotional rollercoaster of caregiving. Although the author's wife had multiple sclerosis (MS), a chronic, disabling disease that attacks the central nervous system, his dilemmas are similar to anyone in the depth of caretaking.

This jewel of a book is filled with useful and practical advice that covers topics from Dr. Rob's personal journey with his wife, Cindy, and their intimate battle with MS. For two decades, the author has immersed himself in the emotional, psychological, and medical research to be the best caregiver he could to his partner. At the same time, he also continued to raise his two children, who were relatively young at the time of their mother's diagnosis. Rob Yonover walks us through a heartfelt journey with ease to understand explanations of the ins and outs of finding appropriate support services, dealing with extended family, and the art of self-care as the primary caregiver.

The advice in this book not only guides you through the challenges but also is entertaining. Dr. Rob's raw ability to take you into the throes of his life as a caretaker, husband, and father is not only refreshing but his story also offers guidance and hope. Reading the researched ideas and the accompanying compassionate story is well worth the limited time a caregiver has on a daily basis.

Turn the page and start on your way to better caregiving through solid advice and this heartfelt personal story. . . .

—Carlyn A. Tamura, PsyD

Introduction

BY DR. ROB YONOVER

As a scientist, inventor, and extreme waterman, I trained myself to analyze all situations and solve any problems in the most efficient manner possible. I had my world worked out, I thought. And then my world changed.

Suddenly, Cindy, my wife, and I were two people who were not only in deep love, but also in deep shit. Cindy was diagnosed with multiple sclerosis. I wasn't going to let this major challenge ruin the family and love we were so fortunate to have—it doesn't come around that easily.

Don't kid yourself, if you find yourself becoming a caregiver, you are in for the biggest challenge of your life, physically, mentally, socially, and financially, that can ultimately rock the foundation of your relationship. This book is my attempt to equip others who face similar challenges in all types of caregiving with some tips and guidelines to make their situation survivable.

—Robert Yonover, PhD

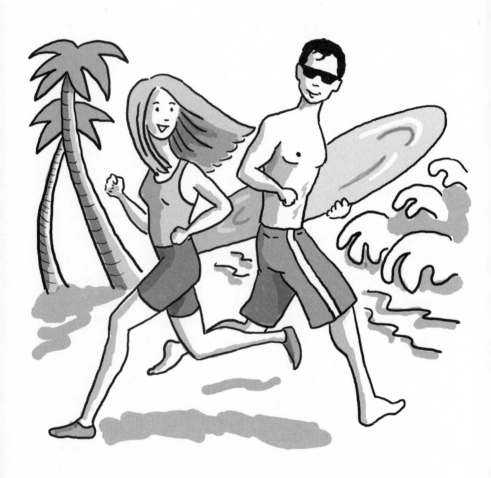

Section 1

Two In Deep

Never above you. Never below you. Always beside you.
—Walter Winchell

The really important kind of freedom involves attention, and awareness, and discipline, and effort, and being able truly to care about other people and to sacrifice for them, over and over, in myriad petty little unsexy ways, every day.
—David Foster Wallace

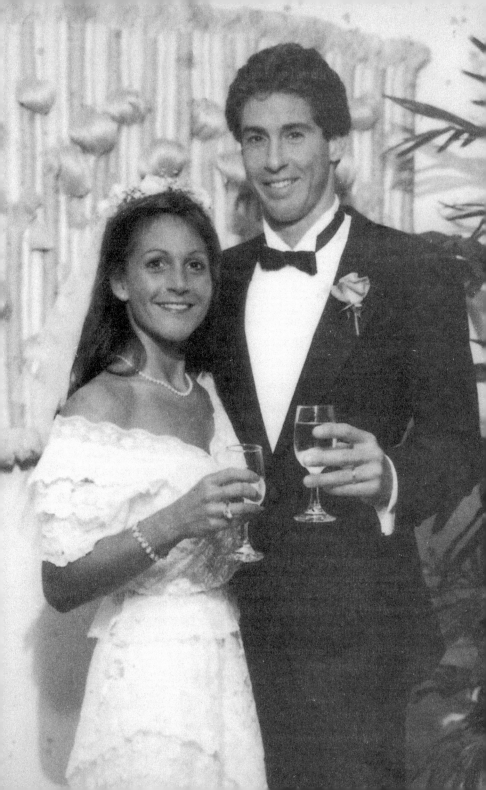

1   Hold On to the Foundations of Your Relationship

Whatever your caregiving role may be (spouse, parent/child, child/parent, friend/friend), I believe it is important to hold on to and respect the foundation and origins of that relationship since in many cases, it will drive how you approach surviving what you are about to encounter.

Happy, Loving Couple

My wife, Cindy, and I were a happy, loving couple with two small children. We had it all. Cindy was my soul mate and the love of my life. We lived on the water in Hawaii. Cindy, with her dark hair, dark eyes, olive skin, and killer body, was as beautiful as the day I first saw her scoff at me from her position of hierarchy in high school. Cindy was "cool" in high school and I was not. She got to hang out on the wall outside of our high school with the kids who smoked cigarettes, and I was banished to the nerdy kids in class or the wannabe jocks on the basketball court. It wasn't until college that I pulled off a miracle and matured enough to capture her fancy after years of being "friends only." Cindy had the brains and toughness to match her looks. She could hang with the guys and was an independent force. We had an incredible relationship that included sex that made the earth move; she was by far the sexiest woman I had ever met.

Prior to having children, Cindy and I lived out our geographic fantasies and made it to the magical places of our dreams: Africa, New Zealand, Costa Rica, and Indonesia, all from our home in the Hawaiian Islands. With a master's degree in counseling and social work, Cindy had ascended to the upper echelon in the Hawaii abused children and domestic violence scene. Her energy was so powerful that she had evolved into part-time lobbying for social causes with the Hawaii legislature, always succeeding in getting money appropriated for the abused children and battered women.

My world was off the chart. I had come to Hawaii to get a PhD in volcanology and was fortunate to be one of a few people in the world to work on ocean floor volcanoes by personally going down two miles deep in the *Alvin* submersible. If that wasn't fortunate enough, I monitored active Hawaiian volcanoes and performed laboratory work at NASA's Johnson Space Center and at the Massachusetts Institute of Technology. The icing on the cake was my patented invention of the See/Rescue Streamer, a revolutionary rescue device that became approved and used by all branches of the US military and some foreign militaries. It saved multiple lives!

At home, things were going very well. Our relationship was perfect and our son and daughter were beautiful and gifted. With both of our careers booming and with my successful home-based invention laboratory in full swing, we had enough money and time to raise our elementary school–aged children firsthand. The mothers in our circle referred to me as

"Mr. Mom," but I pointed out I was actually "Dr. Mom" since I had worked very hard for that title!

I was an avid waterman, which included surfing serious giant-sized waves on Hawaii's famed North Shore. Cindy's passion was long-distance running. She pushed herself hard and was quite an athlete. Her goal was to run the Honolulu Marathon.

During an early autumn marathon training session, Cindy's left leg started to drag a little. That first limp was the beginning.

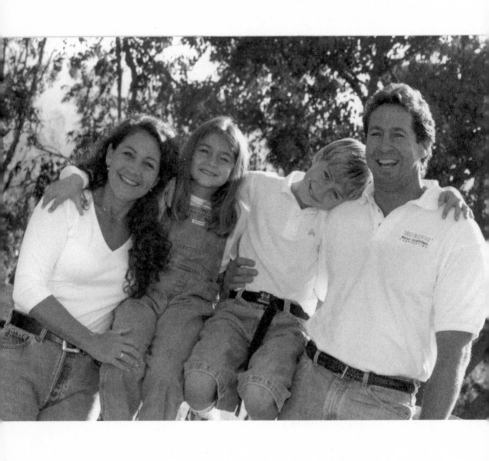

2 Dealing with Heavy News

Brain Stem Lesion

The doctor sat us down and gave us the bad news. Cindy had a lesion on her brain stem. The MRI showed it, and the prognosis of multiple sclerosis was not good. That was a heavy piece of news. After the initial shock, we reflected on how fortunate we were to have had the incredible life we'd experienced up until then, including the fact that at least our children were not sick—that would have been something we could not begin to fathom. We were in our midthirties, and we both had experienced overachieving, exciting lives to date, both before and after hooking up. Being the hard chargers we were, we were not going to take this prognosis sitting down. We were going to fight this illness.

Telling Your Family and Friends

A very difficult task was telling Cindy's family. Cindy was the star of her family and the news rocked her parents' world. They immediately jumped on a plane from Miami and tried to do their best to help us.

It's always hard to be the bearer of bad news; however, this was especially hard since Cindy looked so healthy and perfect. No one believed she would ever get sick, especially at the young age of thirty-six! I am great at rationalizing, so my strategy was always to tell people and try to minimize the horrific aspect of the news by including the positives and potential for her to get better or at least keep the disease at bay. I cited the great progress they were making with MS drugs and treatment and assured people that we were not going down without a fight. Nevertheless, no matter how much you sugarcoat it, the news was not good, and it brought about the full range of responses.

The one thing I learned from telling people bad news is that you have to let them react their own way. You can try to guide them; however, they are going to take the conversation and interaction to a place they feel most comfortable. In a manner similar to the way in which people would later look at Cindy in a wheelchair with a mix of horror or pity, the same thing happens with conveying bad news. It was like going through individual mourning sessions with each person and listening to how they projected their own feelings and fears onto our challenging medical situation. Some people have knee-jerk reactions and want to do radical things to try to save her, while others are just paralyzed by the news and become almost catatonic. You really learn right away what people are made of and what kind of personal trauma and experiences they have gone through themselves.

The good news on this front is that the process of telling people helped us process the news ourselves. At first it is surreal, but after telling family and friends it really hits home, and you are forced to deal with the reality right away. I also personally became empowered by the shock I felt from the reaction from family and friends in that it made me want to survive this ordeal for all of us. I was always a person who liked challenges, especially as an underdog, and this was the ultimate challenge that would test me to my core on all fronts! There was no way I was going to wimp out and let Cindy or our kids down. Game on.

Cindy and I had very different upbringings. I lived and breathed sports, including potentially deadly interactions with nature and severe guy-to-guy personal verbal attacks. Growing up, my buddies and I had cut-down fights for fun on the streets every night. Cindy had three sisters and never competed in team sports, verbal matches, or battles with nature. I was used to pressure situations; she was not. And like all those thrust into the roles of care receiver and caregiver, we had no idea of the pressures looming on the horizon.

Short-Term vs. Long-Term Conditions

Whether you are at the beginning of a battle with MS or another physical problem or you are dealing with the dementia of a family member, try to take the long view. I guess it's a lot like Alcoholics Anonymous, where it's "one day at a time." Each day has its minute-to-minute challenges, so try to pace yourself because you are in for a marathon battle on all fronts.

In our case, Cindy's MS happened gradually, preparing us for the endgame. In the case of MS, it was the loss of mobility, limb by limb, resulting ultimately in complete paralysis and the wheelchair over several years. If Cindy had gone from doctor's diagnosis to wheelchair within a few months, it would have been more devastating. It was much more doable to get used to the limp, the cane, the walker, on the way to the wheelchair. I think dementia and Alzheimer's are also similar in that things may start slow and build to a (bad) climax with time.

Those who become caregivers instantly (e.g., paralysis by car wreck) probably have the hardest time adjusting. Our gradual downward spiral to the wheelchair was more palatable, just like the ten months of pregnancy or the stages in our children's development from baby to toddler to shit-talking teenager to respectable young adult (ha!). Humor and perspective—don't try caregiving without it.

Humor, interjected into situations by me more than Cindy, as I needed a way to survive the day-to-day serious challenges that we faced, was a constant presence in our relationship. It was shocking for people who didn't know us to see how we interacted, with serious black humor and in-your-face banter. It was kind of like *Seinfeld* on steroids—with real issues. Cindy was always a tough character with an excellent sense of humor—we were testing these limits every day. If the public could handle it, we could easily have formulated a sitcom that could really normalize the existence of wheelchair-bound people.

In the early days, it was interesting to note how people physically reacted to seeing someone in a wheelchair. The reactions ranged from people completely ignoring us as we went down the street to over-the-top sympathy—both were a bit of a bummer, but we got used to it. When you coupled the visual with our hardcore bantering, most people just ran for the hills.

I think one of the factors is that people who are not dealing with a serious illness can't even imagine it. People were basically in shock when they interacted with us. Plus, we were shockingly open about everything and left nothing inside our heads to eat away at us. Cindy taught me early on, in the non-MS days, to let all my feelings out and not keep them in where they could become toxic. That was a critical lesson; however, I think Cindy sometimes regretted it, as I don't let anything fester inside me. This led to impromptu arguments and discussions at occasionally inappropriate times.

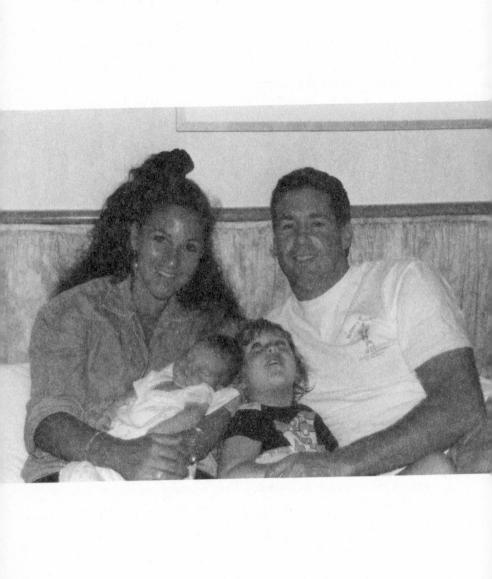

3 Dealing with Daily Challenges

Loss of Mobility and the Dreaded Wheelchair

Cindy and I were in our own fight, fighting off the ravages of MS as it progressively took away her limbs. She resisted using a cane for as long as she could, but needed one to support her right leg that was dragging more and more. Cindy always kept her sense of style and used only a hand-carved cane from Africa. Ultimately, however, she needed a walker to support herself and not fall down while she fought to propel herself unaided.

The thing we fought for the longest time was the dreaded wheelchair. Not accepting it as a tool was getting hazardous because Cindy was starting to fall more and more when only supported by a cane or walker. Cindy was a proud fighter, and she was not giving in to it fast. Another complication was that she was starting to lose the use of her arms—one at a time. She could barely feed herself with her good arm and needed a special spoon she could grip with her weakening hand. The doctor warned us that once she lost her good arm, we were in for an order of magnitude in change in lifestyle, since she would then require massive amounts of care to achieve the most private actions like feeding herself and going to the bathroom.

It had been about a year since Cindy's first fateful limp that signaled the onset of our struggle; however, we were now going deep into the repercussions of her progressing paralysis. There were many challenges to our situation from both of our perspectives. First and foremost were the basic physical necessities that are obvious for a person rapidly approaching complete paralysis.

Cindy's physical needs required that I essentially become her hands and legs. This meant that Cindy, once a proud, athletic, semimacho powerhouse, now had to rely on someone else to do the most basic things. Yet she looked as beautiful and as vibrant as ever.

We scrambled for ways to cope with our changing lives. Not wanting to make a big deal of our difficulties, we went to restaurants or parties early so I could transfer her from her wheelchair to a regular chair or couch so she would be situated before anyone else arrived. Another important factor was that Cindy, and even more so our daughter, are the densest humans I have ever lifted—they both look light, but they are extremely heavy and hard to move. That made my task of becoming Cindy's arms and legs even more challenging on the physical front alone.

Another glaring issue was that I am not the most physically gentle person—I was infamous for breaking things in the laboratory. I have a heavy hand and touch, as I sometimes don't know my own strength. Combining this characteristic with Cindy's increasingly sensitive body conditions made it even tougher to lift and transfer her without hurting her. To add insult to injury, I am six feet one in height, and Cindy is only a little over five feet tall; therefore I had to bend over to do most any physical action for her.

Developing My Feminine Side

Although my feminine side is heavily developed after being raised in a progressive family with a feminist mother, I still was forced to learn the ways of a female. Starting with the basics, I knew what to do with her private parts from a lovemaking perspective, but not necessarily from a sanitation angle—especially given the difference between indoor and outdoor plumbing.

On a practical front, Cindy's physical limitations and my taking on the task of becoming her arms and legs made for some challenging situations—especially when it came to the public bathroom. This is true for any male caregiver of a female patient. The problem was that Cindy refused to use the men's bathroom, so we were relegated to the women's bathroom in public places. This was quite a shocker for a macho guy who had never been in a women's bathroom in his life. I have to say, they were definitely cleaner—women don't miss the toilet as much as men. My strategy was simple when faced with the situation—get in and out in a stealthy manner so the other women didn't know a male was in their bathroom. Typically, we'd roll in and make a beeline for the handicap stall.

I'm sure other caregivers in this situation know how much we appreciate the modified spaces when they are available, and we thank the Americans with Disabilities Act all the way.

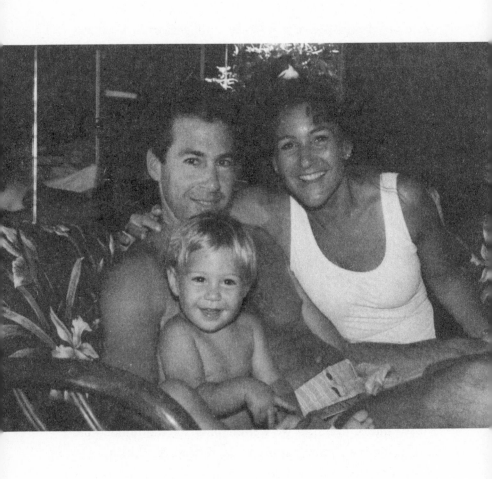

4 Why Me? And the Blame Game

You're in the doctor's office and the news rolls off his lips, "You have multiple sclerosis. . . . I'm sorry."

Cindy's and my first reaction was disbelief. How could that be? Cindy was such an athlete and perfect human specimen, with an impeccable diet on top of that. She'd been a vegetarian for thirty-plus years. Of course, the "why me?" subject came up. We tried not to dwell on it because that will get you nowhere—quickly. We did not know much about MS, so it was pretty scary. What we learned had some encouraging news, such as that the prospects for MS were not that bad unless you had the bad kind. There is the minor type, the relapsing-remitting type, and the primary progressive type, the worst kind. Of course, we were hoping for the minor kind and, being fighters by nature, we were ready to take it on— whichever one she had! We staggered out of the doctor's office with a massive load on our minds.

Many about-to-be caregivers will find themselves in this situation. At this point, I recommend going to a quiet place, preferably a natural setting like the oceans, mountains, or a forest, and try to take stock of your life and review all the things that have gone well for you prior to this shock. The battle you are about to undertake is a long and hard one, and you have to pace yourself. Ironically for us, it was a lot like the marathon Cindy was training for when the first limp struck! We were in a real marathon, with massive things at stake—not just a good finishing time.

The thing you want to avoid, but ultimately is unavoidable for at least a few rounds, is the blame game. Cindy's blame centered around the stress she was under from her high-pressure job as administrator of a major social service agency in Hawaii helping abused kids and battered women. Whether it was the stressful work environment, her coworkers, or just my inability to make millions of dollars that would have enabled her not to work, they were all targets at some point in time. There was even a time when she blamed the physical site where she worked—apparently it was a nasty dump site with the ground being treated with chlordane, a pesticide that is known to cause major medical problems. In fact, this blame may have had some credibility since many of Cindy's coworkers came down with neurological disorders over the next few years, way more than what is considered statistically possible.

The blame game was on, and I had a few blames I threw in the pot, mainly centered on Cindy's diet. Although it was seemingly ideal with the vegetarian slant, perhaps iron and vitamin B were deficient in her body. My strongest blame was artificial sweeteners. The one thing I always hassled Cindy about was her daily intake of multiple diet sodas and using that same artificial sweetener in her hot coffee before she went for a run in the hot sun. That seemed like a chemistry experiment to me.

I think it is slightly therapeutic to play the blame game for a little while. It makes for good venting, a requirement of the battle and journey you are about to undertake if you find yourself in the caretaking position, whether you are the caregiver or the one being taken care of.

Of course we were hoping for the doctor's news to be wrong. In fact it was only ten years later that Cindy finally accepted that she actually had MS. Her situation was a weird one since she only had one lesion on her brain stem and MS implies multiple lesions, as in multiple sclerosis.

I think it is useful to keep a slightly angry edge to give you the ability and attitude to fight off your medical sentence. Cindy was not going to let this beat her and she always had that edge of anger brewing below the surface. I think it provides good fuel to fight the multitude of battles on the horizon for people in our position. The other thing to realize right off the bat is that you and your partner are going to ream out each other, becoming each other's punching bag and pressure release source.

Although it may not be the healthiest thing to do, I believe it is better than letting your anger and resentment stay bottled up inside you, leading to a massive eruption at a later date. As a scientist studying the different kinds of volcanic eruptions, I learned that the ones that build up the pressure result in extremely violent and deadly eruptions versus the ones that erupt all the time and release the pressure constantly—for example, Mount St. Helens's dangerous eruption versus the mellow eruption of Hawaii's Kilauea volcano.

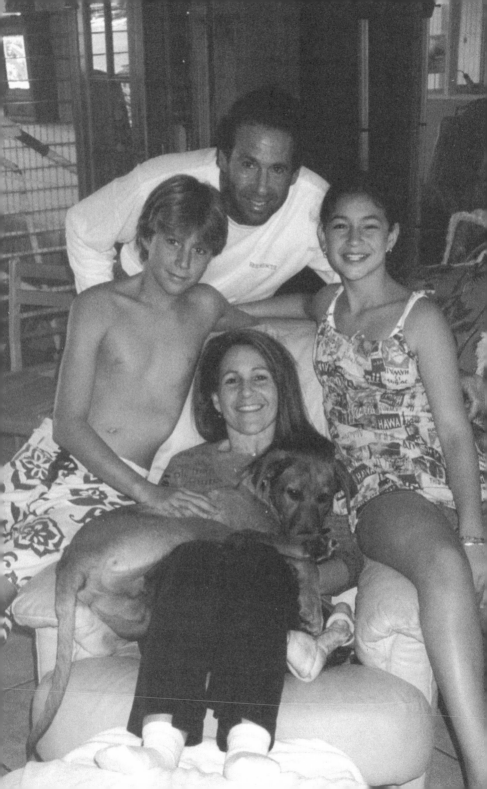

5 Take Stock of Your Ship

You have just been read the verdict—your spouse or loved one requires caregiving, and it is only going to get harder with time as the illness progresses. Now what? The best analogy I can come up with is that a category 5 hurricane is coming toward you. It's time to batten down the hatches, and the worst part is that the hurricane is going to hit you and then, instead of passing through, it's going to hover over you for years! Shocking and sobering news, but it's true!

As a big-wave surfer, rough-water fisherman, and volcanologist, I was used to preparing for storms of all kinds. That gave me the advantage of knowing how to prepare for, react to, and endure a massive storm of any kind.

The preparations needed and the problems I faced are similar to those faced by millions of others. More than fifteen million Americans provide unpaid care for a person with Alzheimer's disease or dementia. The largest proportion of those caregivers is spouses, followed by children and children-in-law and friends. Caregivers need all the help they can get.

Without caregivers, people with debilitating diseases and

dementia would have a poorer quality of life and would need institutional care more quickly, and national economies would be swept away by the advancing demographic tidal wave.

How's Your Ship?

The first step is to take stock of your "ship" before the storm hits. I am using the term "ship" in the broadest possible sense. Your ship consists of your physical plant—your home, car, neighborhood, and all the physical objects/tools in that plant.

Modifications are going to have to be made to your home to accommodate a person with diminishing physical and mental capacity. If you're not in love with your house and neighborhood, you may want to consider moving into a single-story home in an area with shops nearby to minimize the hassle of everyday tasks. Otherwise, you have to be prepared to modify your home, including ramps, stair lifts, grab bars, and other handicapped-accessible improvements. The easier you can make your life in advance, the better. If you live in a remote area on the side of a mountain in a three-story home with tight stairwells, you may want to consider relocating. The simpler you can make the basic everyday tasks like moving around the house or running errands to the drug store will leave you with more time to tackle the harder problems involved with caretaking.

What's the wildlife population like in your home? Are your children young or grown up? Can they be of assistance, or do they require care that will add to your load, especially now since your partner is becoming less able to lend you a hand? Do you live near your children's school or a bus line to make them more self-sufficient? In a strange twist on the caregiving experience, I believe our children gained a level of responsibility, respect, and resourcefulness that was one of the few fringe benefits of having a physically impaired parent— aside from the obvious break of prime parking spot (handicapped) locations (bad half joke).

On the flip side, I highly recommend obtaining as many four-legged creatures as possible, without becoming the cat lady down the street. Although I initially fought the idea of getting a dog, as we already had two cats, Cindy and the kids won out on that argument and finally broke me down. Of course, they promised to clean up after the dog, but that ended on the second or third day—I can't recall exactly. We scored a puppy Labrador retriever that added a ton to my work/responsibility load, which is why I fought it in the first place; however, in retrospect, it was the best move we ever made.

A few years later, someone gave Cindy a yip-yip dog that I also fought against, but again surrendered. In addition to another mouth to feed and rear end to contend with, this dog was a bit of a fu-fu dog that did not help my macho reputation when I walked it around the block; however, we let his hair grow Rasta style, and I got over it. Dogs and cats provide a great pressure release for all members of the family that is essential in the struggle you are about to undertake. Their unconditional love and constant presence with a dog-/cat-tooth smile is priceless, if for nothing else than to provide you with a centering influence on a bad day or moment. They also provided a nice level of security for Cindy when I had to run out to the store and she had to be alone for a short period of time.

Dogs are very intuitive when it comes to protecting someone in their family who has limited ability to protect themselves. The Lab, Rocky, also provided the bonus service of licking Cindy's face in the morning. She has incredibly oily skin, in a good way, that kept her looking beautiful and ten to twenty years younger than her contemporaries; however, it's good to remove the oil for the next layer to come, and Cindy's skin had a nice taste that Rocky and I competed for—he usually won in the morning, and I won at night!

Assess the Mental Health of Your Team

You are about to take on a long-lived journey through a hurricane, so remember to keep your sense of humor, if possible, and your ability to become a lemonade factory (when life gives you lemons, make lemonade…). Look for any little victory you can secure—they will be few and far between relative to the everyday challenges you will encounter, analogous in many ways to child-rearing.

Mental health is probably the most important tool you have in your upcoming battle. Not just your personal mental health, but the mental health of your spouse, children, and relatives. As in an at-sea emergency, figure out which people are stable and can be leaders and which need to be directed and kept calm. In a survival situation, your brain is the most important tool you have. In caregiving, I believe it is the same.

Once you have ascertained the mental health of your team, try to shore up any problems if you can. If your relationship with your spouse had a few sticking points before the illness, they are only going to get magnified heavily after the illness sets in. Therefore, I would recommend going to counseling or therapy immediately after your diagnosis. You need to make your relationship rock solid, and if it is a slow-onset illness like MS or dementia, you have time before the hurricane-force winds really start shaking your house.

I know that most men are fairly reluctant to go to counseling; however, a progressing illness on the horizon is the perfect excuse for guys to get over that macho belief that counseling or therapy is for sissies. Counselors provide a referee and guide for the two of you to hash out your problems. Again, the problems you have before the illness will likely pale in comparison to what you are about to encounter. In fact, as a veteran caregiver, I laugh at the things we used to think were big issues! However, those little issues, if not resolved, can blossom into full-blown infections if you don't deal with them early and often!

Children's Needs

In many ways, our children turned out with skills that are beyond most adults in that they witnessed and experienced a higher level of marital commitment and overall struggle with respect to the physical health, well-being, and financial survival. They learned what it is like to be in challenging situations and the meaning of the word *persevere*. In addition to observing firsthand the strengths, trials, and tribulations of a debilitated mother, they also assisted in her care in many ways. Our attitude was one of acceptance of Cindy's MS condition and full throttle ahead to live a full life despite it. We tried never to let it get in the way of the things we wanted to experience as a couple or as a family unit.

The work ethic was strongly instilled in our children as they witnessed one type of work or another, from making a living to providing care for their paralyzed mother. Cindy stayed completely active in all parental and family decisions and remained a powerful voice and example for the kids to follow. Despite her physical condition, I never discounted her opinion and included her on all major parenting and household decisions. The kids got to experience how, despite her condition, she could remain a strong member of our family, and that was a powerful message.

Cindy and I believed that our children were not the center of the universe. It was the opposite—Cindy and I, the parents, were the center of the universe, and they needed to respect that fact and ultimately work hard to become a member of the ADULT club. The kids had their responsibilities, mainly school, and we, as parents, had ours. We fit the children into our schedule, not the other way around. We were proud when both of our children were honor students and went on to postgraduate college degrees without us ever helping them in any of their studies.

This strategy was even easier to deploy given Cindy's situation and the fact that we were both so fully engaged in battling her illness, in addition to my efforts to make enough money to keep us afloat. They learned very early on that we had no time to deal with their (minor) schoolwork issues and that it was almost an insult to even consider asking us for help. That is not to say we didn't constantly debate them on many of the topics they were learning about or understanding the world and how it works in general. We always had lively discussions and debates on subjects that ran the full gamut.

Assess Your Own Health

One aspect of caregiving that is commonly overlooked is the health of the caregiver themselves. I was informed that nearly 60 percent of caregivers die before the care recipient! That is probably a skewed statistic relative to elderly couples; however, do not discount the toll about to be taken on you physically, as well as mentally and socially.

Take stock of your health right away. Get a full medical checkup, and then look in the mirror. Are you in good shape? If not, you better get in shape fast because it is extremely physically taxing to become the arms and legs of your spouse. It's just like a pregnant woman who has to take care of two people with one body! There are two lemonade-out-of-lemons benefits to getting in shape. Aside from being in better shape and living healthier and longer, the exercise you do to stay in shape will give you that mental health break and a time for you to have some solitude to recharge the batteries.

I personally try to work everyday tasks into an exercise regime, as I actually hate exercising for exercise's sake. By morphing errands into exercise you are creating lemonade out of lemons and killing two birds with one stone. (Are those enough clichés for one sentence?). In the context of caregiving, if I had to go to the store to get Cindy her medicine, I rode my bicycle, or if I had to drive, I parked at the farthest parking stall in the lot and walked briskly to and from the store. I took the stairs if at all possible and always looked for ways to turn errands into exercise.

Aside from animals, my other key calming influence is nature. If at all possible, try to escape to nature for your exercise or breaks. Running errands by walking or cycling gives you a taste of nature and at the same time provides exercise. You will be doing a lot of soul searching and asking yourselves why this illness came to your door. I find that being in the presence of nature somehow puts things in perspective— as beautiful and peaceful as nature can be, it also can be cruel and ruthless. Somehow, your situation fits into the big picture, and perhaps nature can provide insights for you too. From a practical point of view, the fresh air alone is worth the effort. Learning to become one with nature is an acquired taste. I would recommend reading Thoreau or Emerson to get you started.

Manage Caregiver Stress

Among ways to help manage caregiver stress, the National Institute on Aging suggests the following:

Ask for help from family and friends. Specify ways that would help, ask people to take the care recipient for an outing, or make a meal, or visit for a short time.

Focus on what you are able to provide.

Set realistic goals.

Establish a daily routine.

Say no to requests that are draining.

Get connected. Find out about caregiving resources in your community. A helpful website is https://eldercare.acl.gov /Public/Index.aspx.

Look for caregiving services such as transportation and meal delivery.

Check possible programs and benefits available on https: //www.benefitscheckup.org.

Join a support group that will provide encouragement and problem-solving strategies. People in support groups are going through the same things and understand the problems.

Stay well connected with family and friends.

Establish a good sleep routine. Stay physically active. Eat well and drink plenty of water.

Take care of your health. Get recommended immunizations and screenings. Make sure to tell your doctor that you're a caregiver. Don't hesitate to mention any concerns or symptoms you have.

For more information check out the National Institute on Aging website, https://www.nia.nih.gov/health/topics/caregiver-health.

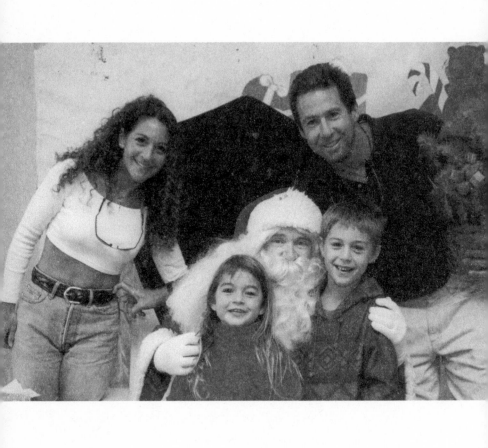

6 Caregiver Mental Health Breaks

As discussed earlier, it is critical that the caregiver is in good physical and mental shape, for without him or her everything falls apart. I was constantly monitoring Cindy's helpers for signs of fatigue, mental breakdown, and all-out violence. Cindy was a tough woman and was used to hanging with a tough crowd. She was a bit of a tomboy, and that is one of the things that I found attractive, especially for the prospect of a long-term relationship. Together, we could be very hard for people to handle or even witness, as we didn't pull many punches during our discussions/arguments. Some of Cindy's caregivers were just completely overwhelmed by the situation, including her personality and our interaction. I closely monitored them and was quick to give them a break or a pep talk, especially the first few days for a new employee, as that was the most likely time for them to quit. Sometimes, it was just easier to let them go and have me take over for the rest of the day (or days) until we could find someone who could handle it. Just like doctors can lack bedside manner and be insensitive to patients, caregivers should probably be schooled in dealing with difficult/

challenging patients (and their partners)—especially the verbal and mental portions of the job.

On the other hand, I made sure to watch over my own mental health, as I was the one with the weight of the world on my shoulders—paralyzed wife, growing little kids, disastrous finances, and so on. I had a few tricks, and the number one thing was always the ability to take a break. The breaks could be physical, like my daily two-mile paddle out into the ocean, or mental, where I tried to watch a movie, preferably foreign or depressing, late at night. Ironically, I found that heavy, depressing movies were actually therapeutic for me, as at the end of the movie I would always look at my situation and say, "At least I am not that guy in the movie starving or having bullets flying at my head!"

It's funny because Cindy and I ended up enjoying the exact opposites in terms of movies. She became a huge fan of rom coms (romantic comedies) and because I set up an office in our bedroom, I listened to many of those as I worked at night. They were perfect for her because they were light and fluffy and reminded her (and me) of what we had together in our love affair. I was barred from watching my heavy movies with her. She couldn't handle them, so I had to move to another part of the house. I guess you have to find out what works for you as an individual and as a couple when it comes to getting those mental breaks and when you find it, keep doing it!

Caregiver Escapes

Caregivers of family members frequently do not get time off. Unless the caregiver mentions it, others simply do not think of it or realize how hard it is for them to get away. The emotional and physical demands involved with caregiving can strain even the most resilient person. That's why it's so important to take advantage of the many resources and tools available to help you provide care for your loved one. Remember, if you don't take care of yourself, you won't be able to take care of anyone else.

Giving yourself a break can help relieve stress, boost your mental wellness, and recharge your batteries. If you can just escape for a little bit, you'll be better able to take care of your responsibilities as a caregiver. Mini escapes can help recharge. So choose what you'd like to do for your escape and work on asking someone like a family member or a community health aide or volunteer to take over while you do it.

Given the physical, mental, and emotional stress of my caretaking role, not to mention the parenting, work, and financial challenges, I learned early on that if I didn't get quality mental health breaks, I would soon be on the watchtower with an AK-47 or just walking the streets of Waikiki talking to myself. Fortunately, we have a townhouse on the water and I am able to jump in the water with my paddleboard and paddle out into the ocean for a couple miles. The roundtrip takes about forty minutes, and it usually delivers a base level mental break. I actually sort through many topics during those forty minutes and have many breakthroughs in my inventing world, as well as my caretaking/parenting challenges.

Every week or so, when things got really heavy, I really needed to get away, and fortunately I pulled it off by going twenty-five miles offshore to Molokai waters and fishing, preferably alone, usually resulting in a clean mental bill of health, plus fish to sell to the restaurants and feed the family and friends. Cindy used to love the boat; however, as her health declined, it hurt her to go over choppy seas, and it's very bumpy in the rough Hawaiian waters. When she couldn't go with me, I tried not to rub in what an incredible trip or experience I might have had. The best way to deal with that was to write up a blurb on my adventure and share it with friends via email.

My life was getting crazy, juggling a variety of tasks that were critical in many ways. Survival became the clear theme of my life—my inventions, my family, my ocean activities, all centered around surviving. I took the Alcoholics Anonymous mantra of "one day at a time" to heart. Ironically, I found myself inventing survival technology, trying to survive Cindy's illness, and doing my best to survive ocean adventures that were taking place in heavier and heavier ocean conditions like extreme rough water boating in the Molokai channel and surfing giant North Shore waves.

Escape into Nature

To keep my sanity, from a physical, emotional, and mental perspective, I countered Cindy's downward spiral by going further and further into nature (the watery kind). I was a big fan of Thoreau and Emerson in high school and recognized early on that nature has all the answers (at least for me), professionally and personally. My escapes to the blue water were getting deeper and deeper.

Living in Hawaii for over thirty years fed my addiction to the water. I am most at home in the ocean, preferably alone or with one or two friends or family members. I have always embraced my primitive side and extending it to the water was a natural. Instead of humans evolving from apes, I see it as the other way around. I think we should devolve back to apes (water apes to be more specific) and have the mix of evolved human and primitive animal. The wildlife I encounter in the blue always seems to have life in perspective, from the whales to the dolphins to the birds.

With all the problems, I wanted that calm and serenity, and the blue always delivers it to me. My comfort level in the ocean enabled me to take on things I only dreamed of as a small child: twenty-foot-plus waves, solo rough water fishing, long-distance open ocean paddling, rough water swimming, and so on. I reached the nirvana of my high school longing days. I got it all—the beautiful wife, living on the water in the islands, surfing the shit, raising a beautiful family, and having a wildly successful scientific/inventing career. The one catch to the story was Cindy's illness and subsequent paralysis. I viewed that as yet another (major) challenge that would make surviving our challenges even more rewarding.

Go to Your Village

Caregiving can be a lonely road, especially when you run out of tasks and even challenges. I found it useful to always get out of our house and try to change the scenery (if possible). Cindy was not very interested in joining groups of other people afflicted with MS, or even elderly people who were physically challenged, as it reminded her of her situation.

I think it is more useful for the caregiver to reach out on their own to support groups or even talk to people who are experiencing similar challenges. I would make it a point not to purposefully approach people in wheelchairs when I was with Cindy in her rolling throne; however, when I was alone I would often approach others in the wheelchair mode and share notes and stories. I found it very useful to commiserate and even jointly joke about some of the lighter moments of the situation. I had a good perspective on the whole situation, and I often would share that with people who may have been on the earlier continuum of their journey. I found it very cathartic and rewarding to help others with the knowledge that I had gained from my ongoing experience (hence this book you are reading)! I felt like we are all in this together, and if the experience I gained from our challenges could be shared with others to help them made the journey and experience, as bad as it may have gotten, to be very rewarding. It was almost like I was meant to help others in similar predicaments because we had survived and even thrived in our struggle.

When Cindy and I where rolling about town, I always tried to connect her with people who were comfortable talking to her and not in shock or pity mode. Children were usually the best because they would look her in the eye and ask her (not her through me) the real questions with no filter. That helped Cindy feel like she was still a viable person (and a knowledgeable, loving parent). Cindy had a connection to children, and perhaps that is why she preferred to interact with them, rather than adults in a similar predicament. Our absolute favorite was children in wheelchairs or similar challenges, as Cindy could share her compassion and general positive energy with these kids, and in some ways it showed them that they could age and still become beautiful vibrant adults, even if they were in a wheelchair!

I think you have to gauge your partner's comfort zone relative to interacting with others for support. I personally like older people, but I could see how older people in wheelchairs could remind Cindy of the inevitable. I think the most important thing is to just get out there. Get out of your house and enjoy your neighborhood and your town. Sometimes the smallest things, like a baby taking their first steps, can provide much-needed distracting joys! The sad thing is that we are all dying, and your partner in the wheelchair is probably going to die first, so get out there and enjoy the world, nature, and even other people. Interesting people, regardless of the physical challenges, can take you on mind journeys as they share their stories and experiences with you. On the flip side, Cindy and I had such an incredible life that we commonly could make people feel better about their situation by sharing ours (the good, the bad, and the ugly)!

The isolation that comes with the job of caregiving can be eased by attending support group meetings with others in similar situations. Connect to the caregiving community. Support groups provide emotional support and caregiving tips, as well as information on community resources.

Online support groups can be very helpful. A possible choice is to find a local support group through a disease-specific organization such as the National Parkinson Foundation. Another possibility is to contact the Well Spouse Association, a national organization that's made up of spousal caregivers coping with a broad range of medical conditions throughout the United States and Canada, as well as a telephone support group and online message board. The Family Caregiver Alliance has a family care navigator tool to help you locate resources, including support groups near you. You can chat online with other caregivers in the same situation on the American Association of Retired Persons website. Eldercare Locator, a public service of the US Administration on Aging, can help you find services and support in your area.

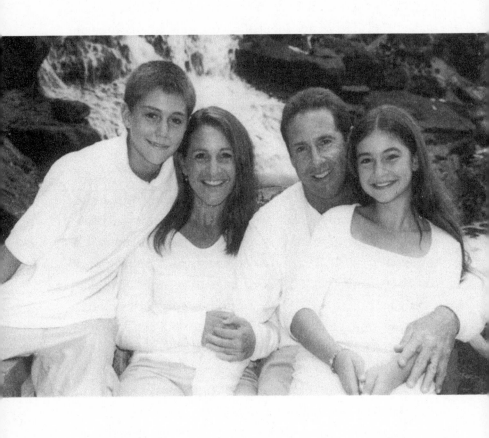

7 Counseling

Even though we thought of ourselves as superman and superwoman, we never hesitated to get professional help when needed. Counseling can help you cope with feelings of anger, frustration, loss, guilt, or work and family demands. Discussing problems with a third party may help with problem solving.

On the counseling front, Cindy went alone and we went together to many therapists over the years, always looking for any insights they could provide (and sometimes they were just simply acting as referees during our grand battles). Cindy was trained as a therapist, so she took great stock in their ability. I wasn't so convinced, but I always welcomed any new perspectives. Having a third party present was very useful to air our complaints and frustrations.

Cindy's solo sessions were very useful, as she would typically be invigorated when she emerged from a session. On the other hand, we were very tough as a couple on therapists, as we were so deeply connected and had been through such difficult times on so many levels that I think we held the record for having therapists quit on us—they just couldn't take it!

We used to laugh about that all the time, as it was usually the other way around with couples and therapists. Nevertheless, I highly recommend counseling alone and together, as even though it may not seem to be much help it is always healthy to air your grievances and try to work things out with a professionally trained third party.

Taking Care of Yourself

The challenge of juggling my newfound role as a caregiver was to make sure I took care of myself. If I got sick or was unable to perform physically or professionally, our entire family would be really screwed.

Given all that is on your plate as a caregiver, you need to find something you can do by yourself or for yourself on a daily basis. For me it is the ocean or the mountains on days when the ocean is unavailable. That is absolutely the key ingredient to my surviving this journey as an unexpected caregiver. Not only is it cleansing, but you get to reengage with your tasks with a fresh perspective and a solo session under your belt.

If you're not into the ocean or mountains, just simply take a one-hour walk by yourself every day. It may not sound like much, but it will help you on both your physical and mental health fronts—the two keys to surviving. You cannot afford to get sick physically, mentally, or emotionally if you are the primary caregiver of a loved one and responsible for the rest of your family. It's just like the flight attendants tell you, put your oxygen mask on first, and *then* help everyone else with theirs!

Value What You Provide

Make sure you value the gift you are providing by enabling another human to survive. Caregivers should be celebrated, and rather than waiting for praise from others, make sure you praise yourself. You are making the ultimate sacrifice, and although the person you are taking care of may not overtly appreciate you at all times (or ever), be assured that they do appreciate you and are indebted to you. This is a critical mindset to have because otherwise you will become unbearably frustrated with the situation. You should be empowered to know that you are stepping up to keep your loved one as comfortable as possible so you can collectively live out your life together as partners. Do not undervalue how powerful this straightforward act can be, and make sure you celebrate it—at least privately.

If you have that attitude, you can remain sane and viable as you encounter the really tough stuff that always seems to be coming around the bend.

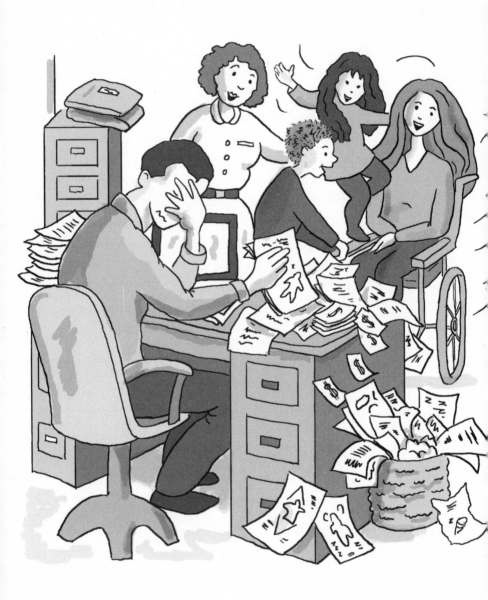

8 Take Stock of Your Finances

Finances—Or the Money Pit

Make sure you are seated before you read this line—having a spouse with an illness that results in paralysis is a financial death sentence. I don't know any other way to soften the blow. Full twenty-four-hour-a-day, seven-day-a-week care costs a fortune—approximately $150,000 (cash out of pocket) annually if you are going to hire private nursing care to come into your home. Other options like care homes or nursing homes are also extremely expensive.

Now that I have sobered you up with that dose of reality, you can attack this challenge like all of the other challenges you will encounter on your journey. Of course, the more you can be your partner's caregiver, the more money you can save. It's frustrating sometimes to perform the tasks of a full nursing staff that would cost approximately $150,000 when all you get is an occasional "thank you." Your rewards are internal and personal; they can't be measured in dollars, especially when you pull off keeping the family together and successfully guiding them through the minefield of a serious illness, and your children not only survive but actually thrive as they mature into young adults and beyond.

Use Your Caregiving Dollars Wisely

I am fortunate to have a career that enables me to work from our home at all hours of the day, squeezing in work and mental health breaks when I can. Keep an eye on the ball, remember to make sure you take mental health breaks, and don't be afraid to hire people to help you—just be strategic about bringing in help. Identify the caregiving tasks that are the most taxing on you, and try to get help first and foremost in those arenas.

For instance, the morning bathroom, bathing, and dressing is the hardest for me, not because of the tasks themselves, but rather the pacing of those events. Remember, I am a macho guy who was thrust into a caregiving role. I am used to bathroom, bathing, dressing events taking minutes not hours; however, it's apparently different for a woman (as I have learned over and over). The other hard part is the reverse, that is, getting Cindy ready for bed in the evenings—tasks made even harder by her having much less energy and patience.

Therefore, if you are on a very tight budget, use your caregiving dollars wisely, and hire people to assist you for the times and tasks that help you the most. Remember, all the pressure is on you as the caregiver to keep it together—you can't get sick, quit, or have a mental breakdown. Start by setting up a budget for your total outside caregiving and always use your dollars wisely and sparingly.

Look into state programs that provide assistance for health-challenged people with financial difficulties. A program in Hawaii, Nursing Home Without Walls, was a great help to me. Programs differ according to the state you live in.

In addition to the obvious huge new expenses you will encounter for caregiving, there are more. You have to allot dollars for medical expenses, prescription drugs, special dietary requirements, wheelchair equipment, home modifications, and so on. Don't be too discouraged, for what you are about to undertake is very rewarding on a personal level, even though you have to step back and/or let a lot of time pass before you can actually see the dividends.

Pick Your Priorities

The priorities in your life have to be radically altered. Remember, the illness is financial suicide, so the goal is to make sure you don't really go bankrupt and make sure your monetary challenges don't tear your family apart.

Money now takes on a different meaning. You have to squeeze pennies out of every dollar. Wasting money on things that are not absolutely required is no longer an option, except of course to splurge once in a while to keep your mental health optimum. A treat may be as simple as an ice cream or an evening out for dinner.

Remember that all we really need as humans is food and shelter, so using that as a starting point in your new life of penny saving can be useful. From a dietary perspective, being forced to skimp on food can actually be a healthy new beginning for you and your family. Eating inexpensive yet healthy food in modest quantities can go a long way to improving your overall health. We could even call this the Hardcore Caregiving Diet. Ha! I was taught as a child to never buy retail and always in bulk—the discount stores like Costco are a godsend—not only for caregiving but also for childrearing. By shopping for and eating the basics, your financial and dietary health can actually improve.

When you combine this with the physical demands of essentially becoming your spouse's arms and legs, your entire body can be transformed. The combination of eating a healthy and modest diet coupled with the rigors of caregiving (mixed in with some mental health calisthenics) have kept this middle-aged man in top physical health.

Seek Professional Advice

There are some ancillary financial benefits you can take advantage of that will help you survive your struggle. First and foremost, confer with your accountant and see what you can do in the way of deductions to your income tax, including home improvements, medical expenses, wheelchair equipment, and so on. You can also research the availability of special programs that may assist you with providing help. The most daunting expense will be your paid caregivers, so anything you can do to lessen that blow will be useful. There are many charitable organizations and volunteer groups that provide free or reduced assistance, even if it's just to provide short-term companionship. This may help clear up a few hours for you to get some more work done or get your mental health break.

9 Seek Ways to Adapt and Still Enjoy Life

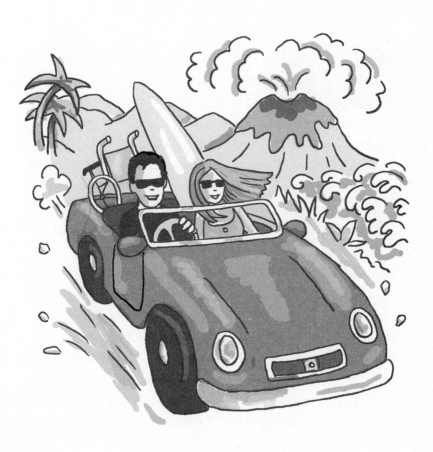

As a caregiver to a disabled, paralyzed spouse, you are essentially morphing your body with your partner's. Therefore, the more ways you can work together, the better. For instance, my home office computer was only a few feet away from our bed, enabling me to work and help Cindy with minimal effort. It's all about multitasking in regard to surviving the financial storm. With a TV (with Netflix?), computer, bed, and bathroom all nearby, you can work, care give, entertain, and powder your nose all at the same time.

Your entertainment budget is one of the things that drops from your priority list; however, by being creative, you can still have a rich cultural and social life. By watching movies or listening to audiobooks together, you can take mind journeys as a couple (or family). In terms of a social life and multitasking, Cindy and I coinvented a cycling system, morphed from an off-the-shelf peddling exercise device combined with a camping chair and creative attachment, that we positioned in the middle of our living room or out on our lanai, depending on the weather, that enabled Cindy to exercise her legs. Wherever Cindy sat peddling in her cycling chair invariably became the gathering place for visitors.

Live by the mantra that your money is reserved for the required things like medical expenses and outside care, and you always have to be conserving money so you have enough to cover yourself. As a caregiver, you are in an epic survival struggle, so don't let something that doesn't mean that much in the overall scope of life (i.e., money) take you down. Save your efforts and struggles for all the rest of the challenges you will face on your journey!

There is such a maze to go through that I recommend early on in the saga that you reach out for advice on financial and legal matters and public benefits. For more details, see section 3, "Reach Out for Help."

Carve Your Joy Niche

Unlike most quadriplegics, Cindy could feel everything. There was a good and really bad side to this. On the bad side, if she had an itch on her toe at two in the morning, I was summoned to itch her toe. Unfortunately, Cindy had a lot of itches. The good side was that she still felt things, preserving the sexual connection we had since day one. We had to be a little more creative relative to her flexibility and positioning; however, the earth still moved, and what I have learned from hanging around psychologists for years is that your sex life is the ultimate barometer for the health of your relationship. If that is the case, our relationship was as solid as a rock.

Keep It Light

Although Cindy had dreaded being dependent on a wheelchair, one of the things we did early on was not make the wheelchair a big deal, especially to the kids. In fact, we encouraged the kids to sit in it and play with it, including using it as a type of skateboard that our son used to "pop wheelies" with by leaning back and riding it on the back wheels only. Of course this was dangerous, but he quickly learned to fall backward on his butt and not let his head hit the floor! Being a practical inventor type with a slant toward efficiency, I learned to use the wheelchair as my main seating tool when helping Cindy out. I could wheel back and forth to feed her food, get the phone, change the TV channel, chase the dog, and so on. On most social events at our house, I had to fight other people, especially kids, for the wheelchair!

Entertainment

When a person becomes confined to a wheelchair, they all of a sudden have much more time to fill because it is much more difficult to travel, go outside, shop, and so on. For Cindy, she explored all the options of indoor living more and more as her illness progressed. At first, she was gung ho to go out and do everything a healthy person can do; however, as time passed, it was just easier to stay at home more.

At first, she started listening to a lot of audiobooks as reading became more and more difficult. I even tried to create a page-turning device for her to use with her one remaining hand, but that didn't work out, as it reminded her of her limitation. Audiobooks were good; however, as with most entertainment, you still need a helper to switch CDs or tapes. Even iPads or laptops still need third-party attention to get started and continue operating. The first sets of books she listened to were self-help books on her illness and overall life perspectives. She then changed to lighter stuff like romance novels. She would be pissed that I am sharing this; however, I think they were very useful because it got her mind in more of the fantasy/exploratory journey mode, and I often became the idealized version of Fabio on the cover of the romance novel (unintended perks for both of us)!

As her illness progressed and access to and usability of the Internet grew, Cindy did a lot of poking around on the web with either my help or one of the caregivers. One word of caution on this was that she did get sucked into a lot of shopping, as they sure do make it easy to hit one button and have a UPS guy pull up a few days later with major damage to the credit cards! I, of course, would encourage her to do nonshopping tasks online. She got very proficient at sending texts via a helper, including several to me a day. Although most were shopping lists, it gave us a nice basis to jointly keep our house operational with food in the cupboards. Depending on which helper was with her, she even would send sexy texts to me that I thoroughly enjoyed—no pictures, but the mind is very powerful.

Some sensory experiences that a care recipient might enjoy include the following:

A hand, neck, or foot massage

Hair brushing

Fresh flowers

Essential oils and fragrances

Stroking a pet or furry toy

Visiting an herb or lavender farm or a rose garden

Rummaging in a box containing photos or personal trinkets

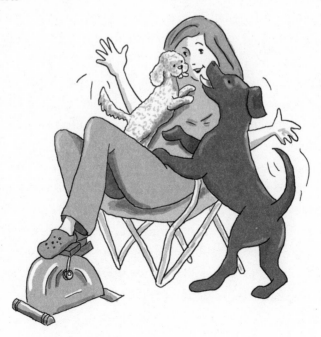

Exercise

Cindy was a workout maniac, and it continued as long as it was possible throughout her illness. She gained both mental health and physical benefits from her crazy lifelong workouts.

Experts advise that exercise is essential for well-being and also helps manage symptoms of MS and dementia. In fact, exercise might even slow progression of MS, according to a 2012 review published in *Therapeutic Advances in Neurological Disorders.*

Exercises to help with balance, strength, coordination, and weight management recommended by exercise physiologists can be found at the National Center on Health, Physical Activity, and Disability.

Doctors' advice is that exercising should be taken slow so as not to strain muscles. Never let a care recipient exercise to the point of fatigue. Forget "no pain, no gain" or "feel the burn." Exercises should start with ten-minute workout sessions and increase gradually.

Make sure all exercising is in a safe place. Avoid slippery floors, poor lighting, throw rugs, and other tripping hazards. Exercising should be within reach of a grab bar or something else to hold on to.

Possible exercises for disabled people, those with dementia, and indeed for mostly everyone, are water aerobics, swimming, stretching, tai chi, and yoga. It's fun to exercise to enjoyable music. Those with dementia may get physical activity and feel useful using soothing skills that have not been forgotten such as washing and drying dishes, sweeping floors, raking and watering gardens, or sorting shells or beads.

Cycling System

Looking for ways to compensate for her loss of motion, Cindy discovered a peddling machine that actually peddles for you via electricity. It seemed like the perfect option for someone in her condition. She was used to working out hard on machines, from her StairMaster workouts at five in the morning while reading a book (before work) to similar rigorous efforts on treadmills. The challenge was how to incorporate this electric foot-peddling machine to fit Cindy's needs.

I took one of our camping chairs that she loved to sit in and strapped her legs to each side of the chair using stretchable belts, resulting in what looked like stirrups from the gynecologist's office (another newly familiar device from my journey as a crossover caregiver). We used Cindy's Crocs (shoes) with straps on them that were able to link up to the straps on the peddling device and presto—Cindy began what turned out to be the first of five-plus years of eight hours a day of "peddling!"

It was a huge breakthrough for her, as it (1) provided the appearance and satisfaction of seeing her legs move; (2) prevented atrophy of her muscles by keeping them in motion; and (3) kept her legs toned, which kept up her smoking-hot body! The only problem was that the devices were not meant to be operated for eight-plus hours per day, and we therefore had to buy a new peddler every few months. We even started packing it in her suitcase when she went to the mainland for trips— you should have seen the looks we got from the TSA agents!

On our lanai at home, we use chairs or stools around the cycling machine to create a party around Cindy, whether it's for a meal, snack, or drinks. By bringing the world to Cindy, we are able to have a rich social life, all for a negligible entertainment budget. We occasionally splurged and bought dinner from a reputable restaurant, instead of the usual bean burritos, and would even light a candle or two. Most of our dates consisted of inviting people over, and I cooked some fresh fish, caught while on one of my mental health breaks, or brought in food, and we gathered around Cindy as she peddled her way through an entertaining evening.

It was also very important for Cindy to stretch every morning to keep her flexible and prevent atrophy. As she got more and more paralyzed, she needed an assistant. Exercise also included getting some fresh air during walks in the wheelchair, boat rides, or a drive in the convertible. Anything that involved motion was good, even though it was not technically exercise.

Mental exercise is equally important, and Cindy's forays into nature were always very useful. Even an hour of sunbathing on the lanai, often topless as a perk, was a valuable interlude. Anything to break up the monotony of being stuck in a wheelchair is extremely valuable, especially if she could be doing something that did not remind her that she was in a wheelchair!

Help Care Recipient Keep a Favorite Activity

The two main areas where I tried to let Cindy keep as much control as possible, as her life and body were essentially out of her control, was managing her staff, including to some extent me, and cooking. Cindy was a fantastic cook, and over the years she essentially taught nearly a hundred caregivers the art of healthy cooking. She would give detailed instruction on how to prepare whatever dish she had a craving for, and that would include the caregiver bringing the half-cooked pan or pot of ingredients over to her to inspect the progress and prepare their next set of instructions. This was an absolute win-win for everyone, as she ate well, her staff was trained, and the sense of accomplishment for her was off the chart.

When you are losing things left and right, it is very powerful to be able to retain a few good things that define you. Her interaction on cooking with her staff also extended to our kids, as she helped both of our kids become fantastic, self-sufficient chefs and bakers. I was part of that training for the kids; however, my specialty was fresh-caught seafood and simple, healthy throw-together meals. Between the two of us, our kids got an excellent start on how to cook and how to eat healthily. We had an ongoing contest in our family on who could eat most healthily that is still ongoing to this day. One of the ways Cindy wooed me in our initial courtship days was with her cooking, and she really never lost her touch, even when she was instructing others to be her cooking hands. That was the basic theme of my overall strategy with her—keep her engaged and in control of whatever she could pull off to keep her mental state positive with respect to being part of our family team.

Many websites offer suggestions for activities a care recipient may enjoy. Here is a sample:

Bake cookies
Make a photo collage
Play and sing music or favorite songs
Pick and arrange flowers
Sort socks
Fold laundry
Eat a picnic
Have afternoon tea

Paint nails
Blow bubbles

Travel Strategies and Fabio

Decades ago, when we moved to an island in the middle of the Pacific, we vowed to get on airplanes all the time and visit our families we left behind and at the same time keep our travel-and-see-the-world quotient as high as possible. Cindy's illness was not going to deter us from that goal. Traveling with a paralyzed person in a wheelchair is no small task. The only perk is that you get to board the plane first (however, you are last on the way out).

The biggest challenge, aside from physically getting her from the door of the plane to her seat, was the bathroom. As everyone knows (especially mile-high club members), airplane bathrooms are tiny and it is very difficult to get two people in there at one time, especially if one of them is a big guy like me. This is where you have to really have your transfer skills down pat, as there is even less room for error. I would have to carry her in my arms to the door and then place her on the closed toilet seat, close the door, and then lift her to get her pants off and proceed.

As her paralysis progressed, Cindy got pretty sick of using the bathrooms on airplanes. She had a few tricks for delaying the use. One was eating salty food (usually nuts) so that she could retain water until we got off the plane and into the airport. We also tended to take shorter travel legs; the five-hour flights were easier than the eight-hour flights. Ultimately, she would wear a Pull-Up (adult diaper), just as a backup. The other little helper was that she always made sure her pharmaceutical supply was at full bore. Everyone knows how uncomfortable airline seats are; imagine being paralyzed so you can't move, yet being able to feel every little pain and discomfort. It was a drag, but we did it over and over.

During one of her trips that I couldn't make, her caregiver was struggling to carry her off the plane when a hunky, long-haired guy from first class offered to carry her. It was Fabio, the Italian hunk of romance novel cover photo fame. That was a lot of fun, and it included a photo in which he looks like he's carrying a toothpick (she was so light to him)!

Despite all the hassles of the airplane portion of our travel, it was well worth it, as we exposed the kids to some great world travel when they were still young and kept in close touch with our families. It also gave Cindy a great take-no-prisoners attitude and provided a sense of accomplishment. She wasn't going to let this minor (really major) issue of paralysis hold her back!

The other thing that is apparent when you travel with a person in a wheelchair is how ill equipped many facilities are for the disabled, especially in foreign countries. Nevertheless, we were creative and persevered as necessary and found it very rewarding to accomplish even the smallest things, like getting to the top of a hill to take in a great view.

Stairs were always a problem when dealing with someone in a wheelchair, and at home we ultimately had to get a stair lift to navigate the stairs from the living room to the bedroom. On the plus side, the stair lift saved us from having to move from our family dream home.

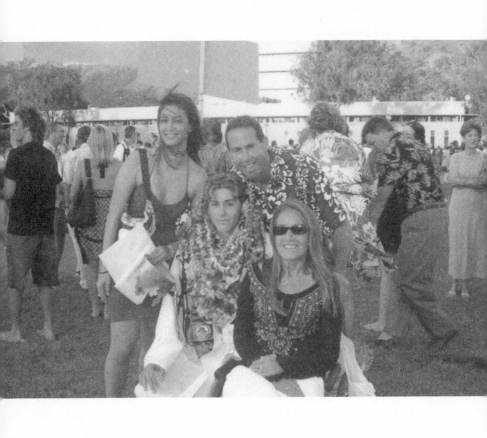

10 Mental Health and Staying Sane

The emotional aspect of Cindy's predicament was the one thing I was not fully prepared for. As the illness progressed, Cindy's resolve weakened and she broke down more often. My family was not known for being a touchy-feely and in-touch-with-your-feelings clan. We came from the "suck it up" attitude. From my grandmother's escape to the United States from Russia to my father's experience in the Depression and World War II, we came from a place that seemed to have heavy drama surrounding us at all times, with no time to get too in touch with our feelings.

Don't get me wrong, my family is very tight and loving, just not in the overt, touchy-feely way. Cindy, on the other hand, came from a family of girls (three sisters) where it was all about emoting—all the time. This was foreign to me, and I learned about it along the way of our journey together. Nevertheless, I was still not completely prepared for the outpouring of emotion that came out of Cindy on an almost daily basis. Deep crying and sadness is a tough emotion to be on the other end of, for me at least. I got better; however, it definitely transferred some of her sadness and frustration when she was depressed and falling apart emotionally. I tried to support her as well as I could, but I usually reverted to a technique I used in child-rearing: "ignore and distract," the two actions that got me through being Dr. Mom.

As Cindy's condition progressed, I tried to provide as many positive distractions as possible. Cindy could no longer do a lot of the adventuresome things we did in the early days, so I tried to make our home as comfortable and as interesting as I could. Fortunately, because we live on the water in Hawaii with an "open-air" house, just being on our lanai and looking out at the water and the passing boats was a great escape. I have often said that all day long we listen to palm trees blowing in the wind and Japanese girls giggling (they were tourists being pulled around on a large, yellow banana raft behind a ski boat). They are two very nice sounds—laughter and wind.

With regard to Cindy, I would first try to acknowledge why she was so sad or depressed and then try to cheer her up by talking about everything we had and not dwelling on the negative of the situation.

The bottom line is an illness like Cindy's rocks you to the core of your being and really brings out how well grounded you actually are. It forces you to deal with feelings and situations you can't imagine; however, as in all difficult experiences, it seems to make you stronger if you come out the other end. I know that my emotional makeup is now much more evolved since I've had to deal with the long-term issues that Cindy's paralysis has brought up. I also think that our children have had life experiences relating to Cindy's illness that have made them better people and that will serve them well in their future lives.

Ignore and Distract

The strategy I developed for dealing with kids applies for all other relationships: ignore and distract. Ignore the bad behavior and distract from the bad or negative elements of life. It was pretty straightforward with young children, as they are easy to "ignore and distract"; however, dealing with adults is more challenging, but potentially as useful.

In having a partner with a debilitating and depressing disease, it is very useful not to dwell on the negative. There is nothing positive to gain from feeling sorry for yourself, except maybe brief periods in which it leads to a good cry to let out your pent-up emotions. I felt my role was to keep Cindy positive with the kick-ass attitude she had had her whole life. This was not the time for her (or me) to get soft—right in the middle of the raising of our young children and faced with daunting physical, emotional, and financial challenges.

If your partner wants to go negative and feel sorry for themselves, you may find it useful to simply acknowledge what they are saying briefly and quickly move on to other, more positive subjects. After all, there is a lot going on that makes it easy to change subjects. Instead of dwelling on the present, it can be good to jump to happier times in the past to reflect on the journey you have had or, conversely, jump to the future and visualize how the kids might turn out and laugh about their little eccentricities and how they might fully bloom when they become mature adults.

We tried not to dwell on the illness itself and the limitations it put on our present life, but rather push through those hassles and focus on the big picture—raising two beautiful, smart, and interesting children and celebrating the fact that we had each other and had survived an incredible journey that was getting even more surreal as we moved forward. Anyone can play a sport when they are not injured. It took real guts and drive to push ahead given the situation we were in. We took great pride in that and found it very rewarding at every step of the way to be pulling off our lives given the "injury" on our plate!

In terms of distracting your partner, there are so many areas of interest you can go into, from your early history to current events, ideas, future wishes, and so on. Assuming you and your partner were a good match from the beginning, there should be nearly unlimited subjects to choose from. Just look at the news, reconnect with friends, or bring up a crazy idea and proceed to have discussions, debates, and even heated arguments. Anything that takes you off dwelling on the disease and your situation is useful. The mind is an incredible tool; it just needs material and data to work with. Take it on yourself to think up good questions that can transfer your partner's mindset by triggering different thoughts, whether they are flashbacks, future visions, or just plain mind exercises and debates. Recall what your relationship was like in the early days and try to go back and capture some of those feelings and themes. By the way, this is not just useful for caregiving situations, but all relationships!

Staying Sane

I knew one of the key things for all of our survival was mental health. As a survival guy, I learned that your most important tool in any survival situation is your brain. We were in a survival situation and our brains remained the most important things. Furthermore, it wasn't just Cindy's brain and my brain that I was concerned with, but I also discreetly monitored our kids' mindsets. After all, they were the most vulnerable in our situation. They were only four and seven years old respectively when Cindy was diagnosed, and we did everything we could to keep them on an even keel.

Our overall strategy was to be very matter of fact about the whole situation with a heavy dose of humor wherever and whenever we could find it. On a basic level, we used to let the kids fool around riding in the wheelchair, and our son, of course, figured out a way to pop wheelies. They would push each other in it and have a good old time with an object that, at face value, was a real bummer to have around if you thought about it too much. I would just downplay our situation and say, "Yeah, Mom just lost her ability to move her legs and arms earlier than us; however, she is still the same on all other fronts."

Along those lines, Cindy hated when people assumed that just because she was in a wheelchair, she could no longer think for herself, and ask me what she wanted instead of just asking her! The other thing we both hated was the pity looks. Some people are better than others in terms of reacting to people with noticeable physical challenges. You learn pretty quickly, usually in a glance, the people who can handle it and the ones who cannot.

It was an ongoing struggle to keep Cindy's mental health and attitude in the positive sector. It was easy for her to get down on her situation; however, I constantly reminded her of all she had relative to what she lost. Ultimately, you cannot convince a person to feel better about their situation; it has to come from within. Cindy was a tough, competitive person, and I played into that by not overly showing sympathy for her. I used to tell her to call her parents or sisters for sympathy and that I was her partner in crime and she needed to suck it up to move forward on our journey. She bought into it because she still had a thirst for life and she wanted to be there for our kids. I used to tell her not to worry about me. I can take all the hits anyone can dish out. However, I also assured her that I was not going anywhere and would be her partner all the way to the end. I think that gave her great confidence that she could absolutely rely on me moving forward, putting her mind at rest relating to having unknowns about her future care.

From my mental health perspective, it always came easily and naturally for me to step up to the plate for her no matter how hard it got, and it did get incredibly hard on many fronts. I was at peace with our situation, and I never felt sorry for myself (or her). It was just the luck of the draw that she got sick (and old) earlier than me. That is how I viewed it and that attitude fit well into our overall strategy of getting married and growing old together. The truth is that up until her diagnosis at the age of thirty-six, we had the perfect lives—children, careers, friends, family, travel, education, professional achievement, and so on. We felt that even though we were in our midthirties, we had lived incredibly full lives already. That helped us in the years to come, as we were both mega overachievers and fortunately had fulfilled all of our dreams and wishes by that early age. I think this enabled us to deal with the challenges that were to come our way.

11 The Social Aspect

The social aspect may be the most important part of the mental health sector of surviving a situation like ours. Although we commonly bowed out of many invitations that she wasn't feeling up to, we never missed any of the happening events, including many boat trips and outdoor activities. Our strategy for parties was to arrive early and take along her camping chair or scope out the most centrally located and comfortable chair at the event. I would set it all up and then transfer her to the seat with or without the wheelchair, and in all cases, stash the wheelchair once she was situated. That made for a much better event as the elephant in the room (the wheelchair) was nowhere to be seen. Cindy was always so hot looking anyway that when she was seated in a chair, you could barely tell that she had any physical challenges and people thought it was romantic that I would be feeding her grapes by hand individually.

As a result of the illness, Cindy had limited energy at times, and therefore we would carefully pick and choose the events we wanted to attend. Of course, it was very easy to back out of events if she wasn't feeling up to it, and no one would mind.

We did that a fair amount to save our energy for social events we couldn't miss. I think it is critical for people in wheelchairs to be taken seriously and not pitied. Cindy was always very outspoken, and that never waned. As her voice got weaker, I became her translator and megaphone. Her self-worth was preserved by keeping up her interactions on all levels, and by being at events with the wheelchair stashed, it was like she was just a regular person, not a disabled, ill woman who needed sympathy!

Visitors: The Good, the Bad, and the Clueless

Although Cindy's parents were put in a terrible spot, having a daughter who becomes paralyzed from MS, they were good about making sure they would come for visits as much as possible. Cindy would often be nervous in the early days, as she worried about how they would react to her appearance; however, they took our lead, and we pushed forward and had great quasi-normal times during their visits. We always went out for a good meal with the entire family at restaurants with tablecloths, and that was always fun.

What people didn't see was that although Cindy was absolutely fantastic in a social setting, restaurants and parties, the meltdown afterward backstage was tough as she had saved all her energy for the event and was completely drained by the end, when I had to get her up the stairs to bed. That was hard but worth it because the upside was so good.

We didn't really have that many "bad" visitors; however, some people just didn't have a clue and were not sensitive to Cindy's limitations or even desires. They would try to pressure her to go on hikes or go boating when she just didn't have the energy sometimes, and they didn't realize the load it would put on me. Another faux pas was trying to get me to split off and go on adventures with them and leave Cindy behind. I figured out early on, and in any relationship, that you can't have more fun than your partner, and that was even more valid when one of you is in a wheelchair.

Overall, many of our pre-MS visitors just simply withdrew from visiting or, in many cases, staying in touch. We understood, as it was so awkward for people who are not accustomed to dealing with a declining person in a wheelchair. Most people don't know what to say or even how to look at a physically challenged person without giving her the pity look (that Cindy so hated and that ultimately made her go out less and less in the waning years).

There is definitely a learning curve for interacting with people with medical challenges, and unless you have had some experience, it is probably really difficult, especially if you don't see the person often and then you see them and they have declined even more rapidly.

Kindred Spirit—Louie Zamperini

People came and went during our MS journey, but when Louie Zamperini arrived, the world moved for Cindy. Louie was lost at sea for forty-seven days and then in a POW camp for two years during World War II (see the books *Unbroken* or *Devil at My Heels* or the movie *Unbroken* for reference).

I met Louie through my See/Rescue Streamer invention (Louie: "Where were you fifty years ago when I needed you?!"), and he and Cindy just absolutely hit it off. Louie's trials and tribulations made it easy for him to relate to her, and Cindy, of course, respected the massive journey he endured. He admired her strength and perseverance, and that is saying a lot coming from him!

Louie was also a very spiritual man and enjoyed praying for Cindy. One time during an intensely physical and mental praying session, Louie broke into sweat and actually had to go back to his hotel room to go to sleep afterward, as it took so much out of him. It was incredible to watch him give his all to try to help her get better, or at least feel better and push ahead. Just by chance, Cindy's sister took a photo during that interaction and the picture came back with a white globe-like structure hovering over the two of them. As a scientist, I have to conclude it was a chance lighting blip; however, it sure looks otherworldly (and none of the other pictures had it)!

In the same vein as my watching depressing movies to make me feel (relatively) better about our situation, it was so uplifting to have a person who had gone to the absolute worst place in life and come back, and even forgiven his torturers, present himself with such grace and generosity. I think it put a lot of things in perspective for Cindy and me. I will never forget his commitment to Cindy and his never-ending humor that always lit up her magical smile!

12 Chasing Rainbows

Dead Man Surfing

When Cindy was first diagnosed, our initial reaction, aside from denial, was to get to the best experts in the world so they could advise us on the state-of-the-art medicine and treatment.

We were put in touch with an MS expert in Colorado, and Cindy began taking trips over there. Among other things, he suggested she move to a cooler climate. This began round one of many battles to find the proper type of treatment and decide which dreams to chase.

Cindy's sisters lived in San Diego, and that became the target destination. I felt that San Diego in summer was hotter than Hawaii. In Hawaii, we lived on a bay, an island within an island, that was so breezy and cool at night that you needed to sleep with a comforter year round with nothing more than a ceiling fan spinning over your head.

I tried to hold my tongue as much as possible; however, I ultimately lost out. Cindy went to San Diego and put money down on a house. I have to say that this was one of the most depressing times in my life. I was forced to choose between the life we had built in Hawaii for ourselves and our family, and what I knew would be a fruitless move to a place that was only marginally cooler than Hawaii. I went along with it to support Cindy and referred to myself as "Dead Man Surfing" as I lived what I thought were my last few weeks of our Hawaii life and saying goodbye to the friends and professional contacts we had built over the years in the islands.

When the deadline arrived for selling or renting our waterfront townhouse in Hawaii, I went for what turned out to be a brilliant move in this chapter of the saga. I took Cindy out on our boat into the ocean behind our house. Here, in the warm tropical Hawaiian waters, she could still pull off her favorite physical activity—topless snorkeling with the fish and turtles. The water was crystal blue that day, and the fish seemed to swarm around her telling her not to go. She came out of the water and back onto the boat with my assistance and uttered the words that I will never forget, "I can't leave!"

We were still in the early stages of our battle with MS. As Cindy's situation progressed, being the fighter she was she tried every imaginable form of medicine or help that could possibly make you better. She did the ABC's of MS treatment that included injecting herself with a shot every day, and she even tried a special chemotherapy that almost killed her. Unfortunately, nothing in western medicine seemed to help. That only left eastern medicine, holistic approaches, and some questionable treatments.

From my perspective, it was difficult to ever question anything she would try, regardless of the price to our savings or to the family. I did not want to be the one that prohibited her from trying something that might make her better. In this matter, Cindy held the trump card. I would, of course, question everything, for example, trips to specialists in Colorado, moving to colder San Diego, and so on; however, I would never stand in her way, and there was still more crazy stuff to come.

This all took an incredible toll on our financial solvency and, at times, our relationship. We lived in one of the highest-cost-of-living places in the country, and this was coupled with the fact that Cindy used to make a good salary before she had to stop working, and she now required 24/7 care. Despite the fact that I performed sixteen to twenty-four hours of the help per day (for free), it still cost approximately $50,000 alone for only eight hours a day of private nursing care to give me an opportunity to pursue my work and take a mental health break. That alone is a $150,000-a-year turnaround—from Cindy making $50,000 a year to spending $50,000 a year on help and another $50,000 on her medical requirements. I understand how many families with a serious and longstanding medical situation go bankrupt.

Israeli Dream

Among the rainbows Cindy chased over the years was a Russian acupuncturist living in Israel, who was supposed to have helped someone Cindy's family knew with MS. From day one, I always thought this was a stretch. I knew Cindy responded well to acupuncture from a Honolulu acupuncturist who relieved some of her pain. Also, knowing that the Chinese, where acupuncture originated, were quite frugal people, I concluded that acupuncture had to be viable because the Chinese would not be getting ripped off for thousands of years! However, relieving pain and curing MS are two hugely different things. I am also skeptical of so-called "healers." If you are a healer sent down by the gods, then why do you charge money, and so much for that matter? Nevertheless, although I made my objections known, I did not stand in Cindy's way of chasing her cure.

It started out with her going to Israel for a few weeks at a time, every few months, along with a bag full of money for the "healer." The bullshit was that she seemed to get better when he worked on her in Israel and worse when she got back. Can anyone say "placebo"? Finally, Cindy made the stand that she was going to move to Israel for a year and give it a shot and she was going to take one of the kids with her. This I fought tooth and nail, but once again I could not stand in the way of her idealized "cure."

Given the ages of our kids, we thought it would be easiest for our daughter (third grade) to go and that it might be a good experience since she was going to attend the American school in Tel Aviv with kids from all over the world. This move hurt and almost spelled the end of our relationship. However, once again I hung in there and kept my eyes on the prize of keeping the family together. My son and I visited them in the summer, halfway through this experience. I gave a briefing to the Israeli Air Force on my See/Rescue Streamer invention, and we got to see a lot of the historical sites; however, the divided family dominated my mindset.

One of the big events was the showdown of when I was going to finally meet the "healer." Of course, he must have been freaking out, knowing he was bilking us out of thousands of dollars. When he showed up at the door, he had his machine gun in hand! That was awkward. The tragedy of 9/11 saved us from enduring more of this Israeli craziness, as once the World Trade Center got hit, I was on the phone to Cindy to get her and our daughter out of the crosshairs. Cindy wanted out of there by then also, and that gave us an excellent reason to go.

Don't get me wrong. Israel is full of interesting people and places, and it was a fascinating place to visit; however, from our family perspective we had to reunite on Hawaiian grounds. A footnote is that my son and I did get to surf over there, and wouldn't you know it, they even had better waves than Miami, where I started surfing!

Quacks 'R' Us

After Israel, and with Cindy still grasping at healing straws, she continued to try anything and everything to stop or reverse the physical tailspin she was in. Cindy was always in touch with her mystical side, including consulting with psychics over the years, a direct conflict with my "prove it" scientific mind. The one proof or coincidence that did occur was that in the year before we had our son, a well-known Vietnamese psychic told Cindy that we would have a blond baby boy in May. We weren't even pregnant, and the psychic knew that both Cindy and I had dark brown hair! That was pretty spooky, as our son was born in May and had blond hair! I still can't fully explain that one. Aside from that fluke, I question all the other "healers" she put to the task over the years (all for money of course). This drove me crazy, as my hands were tied in regard to not blocking her attempts to get better, coupled with the ultra frugality required of me as her income disappeared and her medical costs skyrocketed!

Among the healers was one guy from Florida who would lift and drop her wrist on her belly like a human ouija board to tell him how to advise his client. That would have been unbelievable and laughable if it hadn't cost me thousands of dollars! Then there was the healer who used tiny thirty-dollar vials of oil. Drops were placed in between her toes and behind her ears to initiate healing. Thirty-dollar vials as big as my pinky! There was one healer who used a method based on some actual science and medicine. A stem cell implant was performed on Cindy in Las Vegas (of course) that consisted of taking stem cells from the placenta of trailer park women who had just given birth. The stem cells were rushed to Cindy waiting in the "doctor's" office, a slit was made in her belly, and the stem cell material was placed inside and sewn up. It seemed like quasi science to me until, after her second multi-thousand-dollar implant, we saw the guy on CNN after he got arrested. Un-fucking-believable!

Cindy still tried her best to find that miracle cure. Her next attempt, which of course drove me crazy, was a Vietnamese healer who performed some crude acupuncture on her and appeared to become possessed by a mystical spirit that empowered her with great healing abilities. Yeah right. I was numb to it at this point. I went along with it because whatever gave her hope was something that I couldn't deny her. I knew that if it were me in the wheelchair, I would be trying everything possible also—probably more on the scientific side than the mystical one, but that is just me.

13 Frustration and Loss

It seems that in a fashion similar to childbirth, a major illness rocks people to their foundation. It's hard to explain, except to state that I have seen some very strange behavior by people whom you thought you knew well. The sight of seeing someone you know in a wheelchair brings out emotions, and/or the lack thereof, that you are not expecting.

It was always amazing to me how people reacted to seeing Cindy in a wheelchair. There is always a range of reactions: ignore, pity, be overly nice, and so on. Once we had become more accustomed to Cindy in a wheelchair, it was not big deal for us; however, the same couldn't be said for her friends, family, and acquaintances.

To Cindy and me, not much had changed—we were still the same people, we were just dealing with the major inconvenience of her not being able to move for herself. It is easy for me to see this since I have the perspective of being part of the team with the disability versus the one looking in on another couple with the situation.

The frustration and sense of loss for Cindy was massive.

Not only did she lose her ability to walk, but she also lost a lot of her friends—they were still her friends, but the closeness kind of dried up. People were cordial and polite, but the bottom line was that they didn't really know how to act and were uncomfortable being around her given her situation. Of course it didn't help that we continued to escalate our bickering. We both needed to vent our frustrations, and the closest target was each other. This was healthy to a point; however, it absolutely freaked people out, especially people who didn't know us well or had just met us.

Cindy was always an "in-your-face" powerhouse, which was part of her attraction; however, we both turned it up a couple of notches, and people couldn't handle it, even though it was still grounded in our love for each other and our long history of essentially being soul mates. Being friends for five years before we ever started dating made us very close as friends first and enabled us to survive all the shit that was thrown at us. The problem was that the fireworks and shrapnel coming off of our interactions were viewed as too dangerous for most people to be around. The loss of companionship to Cindy was hard for both of us.

Six-Day War, 2012

The culmination of Cindy's illness and downward spiral led to her essentially having a nervous breakdown and committing an atrocity against our family that I believe was a cry for help. After arguing hard for months with no letup in sight (even therapists couldn't help—a few actually fired us because we were too much for them) Cindy decided to take legal action against me.

I knew she was talking to lawyers; however, I dismissed it as therapy for her and did not think she would follow through.

However, she did. She filed for divorce. This was a huge mistake on many fronts and alienated her family, including most importantly the kids, and caused havoc with our friends.

I took it in stride and prepared to deliver her wish in court, although what she thought was going to happen and the reality were going to be completely different. Against advice from friends who said I should let her follow through and get divorced and go to a nursing home, I fought once again to keep the family together, because as mad as I was at her, I could not abandon her. I was still in love with her and I wanted to keep the family together at all costs.

The judge gave us an hour to reach an agreement before we ever had to go to court, and we reconciled, thereby having the whole action dismissed and keeping this six-day war to a minimum. From then on, it was damage control, and I worked hard to get people to forgive her (and I was first, although I still am mad at her for pulling that trigger, even though she was a sick and desperate woman at that point). Years have passed now and we have buried that event, even though I am continuing to perform damage control on many related fronts.

Bub and Lovie Sitcom, 2015

Cindy and I are essentially living in a black humor sitcom. We are at each other constantly, yet we are deeply in love. We have coped with this situation. We remain together after thirty-three years, from when we first were irresistibly drawn together (after she was no longer an untouchable in high school). As we both approach our midfifties, she remains the sexiest woman I have ever known, even in the wheelchair. There was no one more beautiful, sexy, vibrant, feisty, powerful, and able to hold her own with the boys. Cindy returned to working, from home, on social issues with the Samoan community in Hawaii. I have continued with my survival inventions. We have raised two incredible children who have both graduated from college with master's degrees.

We are in this together and always will be. I have to end now because I am being summoned to the other room—it appears that Cindy needs to itch her nose, and I am just the guy for the job.

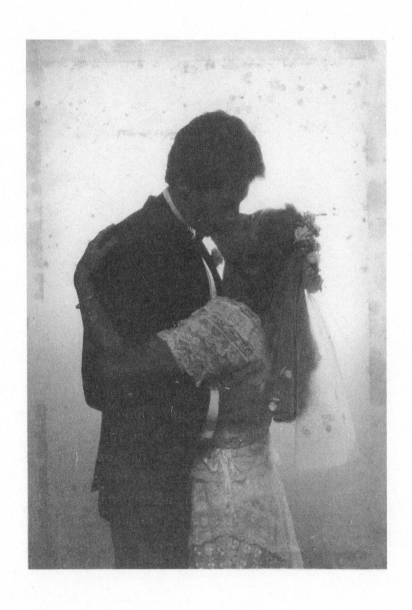

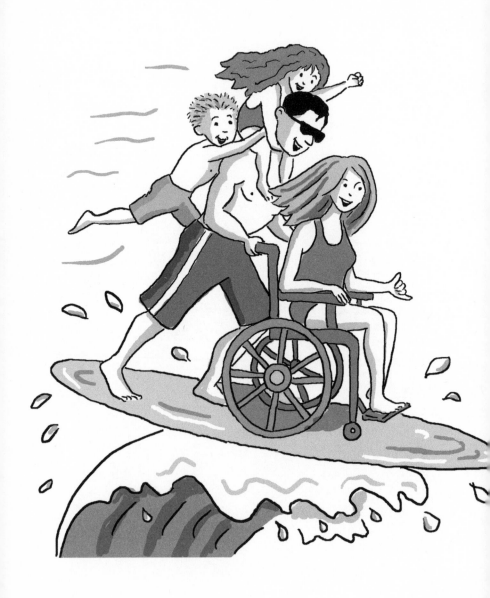

Section 2

Basic Tasks

Stop over-loading yourself with numberless tasks. Give time to yourself for rest and positive deliberations. You can't think better and plan better when you are under stress!

—Israelmore Ayivor, *Daily Drive 365*

We can easily manage if we will only take, each day, the burden appointed to it. But the load will be too heavy for us if we carry yesterday's burden over again today, and then add the burden of the morrow before we are required to bear it.

—John Newton

14 Gut Check and the Daily Challenge

Are you going to be able to handle the basic tasks that make up day-to-day living? Believe me, there are a lot of them!

What are we made of deep down? Can we survive a traumatic challenge? I guess no one really knows until it happens to you. I thought I was tough, but I never prepared for something like this. My immediate reaction was one of commitment, "till death do us part." I was deeply in love with Cindy, and she was the mother of our children. Everything in my gut told me to persevere—at all costs. There was no way I was bailing out.

In a strange way, the overwhelming odds of the challenge drove me to engage head-on with all the personal, emotional, physical, and financial issues. This would be my ultimate underdog challenge.

I had major deficiencies in the caregiving world—I was a macho guy who never took care of people, let alone having to essentially become the only working extension of a woman's body. I would have to transform my personality from a macho "MacGyver" into a cross between "Mr. Mom" (or "Dr. Mom," as my friends called me) and "Nurse Betty." There was no manual to instruct me on how to take a woman to the bathroom and/or change tampons—just Cindy communicating instructions to me!

Trust Your Instincts

With basic tasks, in a manner similar to child-rearing, I found it most useful to trust my instincts. Even though I was a macho guy, I did have deep-seated nurturing qualities that really came to the surface when we had babies. If you don't know how to do something and have never been instructed in that arena, you just proceed slowly and observe how it's going as you move forward. In other words, read the data as it comes in. If you are doing something that hurts the person physically, try a different approach. Communicate back and forth until you reach a process or method that works for both of you, and remember that for the next time.

I think we all have the capacity to be caregivers; it is probably just more deeply seated in some people than in others. When you see a person in need, your natural instinct is to try to help them. The same thing applies to your partner. You have to overlook the trivial issues in your lives and focus on the fact that this person that you deeply love is in deep shit and needs your help. My instinct to help kicks in once I let go of the tit-for-tat bullshit of everyday life and the minor hassles that people experience on a daily basis.

One thing is for sure, an MS diagnosis of your partner, and any other terrible, debilitating diagnosis, really puts life into perspective—especially when kids are involved in the mix.

Feeding

The one thing that Cindy never lost was her ability to chew and swallow, and thus eating became one of the real joys of her life, especially as the disease progressed. One of the doctors early on told us was that once she lost the motion of her last good hand, it would bring on the challenge of someone having to feed her. This was a major emotional challenge as the last few days of feeding herself grew to a close. I tried to keep it light and tell her that she was like Cleopatra and her entourage would feed her grapes by hand and fan her to keep her cool. That only lasted for a few laughs.

In addition to becoming one of the last real physical joys for her, meals became very drawn out as her chewing became weaker. I used to count 40-plus chews per bite to grind the food up small enough for her to swallow and digest. That was hard for me as I was a lifelong food inhaler. It sure taught me yet another lesson on patience. Cindy loved to eat, and I would either prepare or secure whatever food cravings she would have. It was like she was in a perpetual state of pregnancy relative to food cravings, and I was glad to accommodate her on this, for I knew it was pure joy for her. She never lost her taste buds or sweet tooth. She was famous for devouring the icing on a huge Costco birthday cake (vanilla or chocolate, both did the trick). We had many birthday party–like deserts, and I even took to scraping the icing off the cake and freezing it for future sessions. Amazingly she never put on weight.

I think when a person loses the ability to move their body, you have to try help them compensate for that loss by enhancing things they love to do or experience—eating things you love being one of the easiest to perpetuate. By the way, it wasn't just sugar and sweets, as Cindy kept up an incredibly healthy diet for many years, including fresh fish and veggies in keeping with her vegetarian (no land meat) diet.

Suggestions from the National Institute on Aging, https://www.nia.nih.gov/health/healthy-eating, include the following:

Choose nutrient-dense foods. Provide a balanced diet with a variety of foods like fresh vegetables, fruits, whole grains, low-fat dairy, and lean protein meat and fish. Avoid calorie-dense foods with little nutritional value like potato chips, sugar-sweetened drinks, soda, candy, baked goods, and alcoholic beverages.

During the day, offer small cups of water, soup, or milkshakes and smoothies.

Watch for problems that may cause lack of appetite. These may include teeth problems, difficulty with chewing or swallowing, medications, lack of exercise, and a decreased sense of smell and taste.

Serve meals at specific times in quiet surroundings with simple table settings. Avoid new routines.

Be flexible and patient. Give the person enough time to eat.

Respect personal food preferences.

Eat together and try to make it an enjoyable experience.

Sleeping

Sleeping is a tough one, as it affects both parties heavily. To start with, Cindy ultimately was paralyzed with full feeling. Scratching an itch on her toe at three in the morning was a task that she could not complete. I was the official itch master. That has to be one of the worst feelings, to have an itch that you can't get to, similar I guess to having a cast on your arm.

Fortunately, I am able to wake up easily and more importantly go back to sleep easily. (This also helped immensely during the baby phase of our children.) Once again we had to be creative to survive the sleeping aspect of our caregiving challenge.

I guess you never realize how many times you move and adjust your body, until you have to ask someone else to do that for you. For example, here is an overview of the tasks and moves required just to get her comfortable in bed: roll wheelchair to edge of bed; position legs at perfect angle; move hair to left side of shoulder; cross hands over lap so they don't tangle upon transfer; pull pants down over shoes and socks; lift Cindy up and pull pants out of ass; twist and place on bed; unlock wheelchair legs and push wheelchair out of the way; swing Cindy onto bed while supporting her neck and head and not letting her shoes hit the bed; hold up legs and remove shoes; lay Cindy on side, place one leg over the other; remove scrunchy from hair; twist her hips and place one arm in a fist near her crotch and the other straight out on the bed; pull her butt out and push her over to expose her spine and backside toward me; turn on "thumper" hand-held massage wand and proceed to push hard and massage her from the spine downward to ribs to upper back to butt, thighs, and finally, feet—making sure to go from the tip of her toes to the back of her heels; push head down a few inches and pull pillow down under face; insert fingers under head to straighten ear and earrings; pull pillow out of face and eye; watch TV for thirty minutes, then turn Cindy on her back to fall asleep, consisting of aligning her straight in bed; pull butt down; pull shirt down in back and in front; pull shirt out from elbow; place hands crossed over crotch; pull pants down over feet; lower feet to hang one inch over posturepedic bed pad; turn feet outward and place blanket in between feet to keep them angled outward; pull covers up to under chin; blow nose; wipe eyes with tissue; straighten pinky; pull shoulders out individually; repeat as necessary, including the dreaded "I have to go the bathroom again" where the whole process has to be repeated!

Aside from itches and insects, our two biggest challenges were in the physical realm. Cindy liked a soft mattress, and needed it as the bedsore issue became more prevalent, and I like a hard mattress. I solved the problem by inserting a thick piece of plywood under my side of the supportive bed pad. It was great until an unknowing family member or visitor jumped on my side of the bed and got a good, rigid surprise.

It was critical for her to get her sleep and she was a light sleeper so it was even more important for everything to be just right for her. The thing I disliked most was that she enjoyed having the TV on all night. It started with her waking me at three in the morning to turn the TV on when she couldn't sleep, and it evolved into having it on all night. I can't sleep if I have CNN droning on in my ear. Fortunately for me (in this case only), I have a minor hearing deficiency in one ear so I was able to sleep with my good ear on the pillow and thus muffle the CNN droning. As long as I couldn't hear what they were saying, I was able to sleep.

Once again, we took the challenges and needs presented us and worked with what we had to solve the problem. Cindy having a good night of sleep was crucial for her overall health and the stress level of the next day. Even though we were probably better off, in theory, sleeping in separate beds or rooms, I couldn't leave her alone, as she would get nervous and I didn't want to leave her. We just had to get creative in solving the problem.

When I would leave town, we would have helpers sleep in a separate room and use a baby monitor. That worked OK, but Cindy really never could sleep well like that. We were so used to sleeping together that it was a major strain for her to be alone, especially in her vulnerable state of immobility.

Suggestions from the National Institute on Aging website, https://www.nia.nih.gov/health/6-tips-managing-sleep-problems-alzheimers, include the following:

Maintain regular bedtime routines.

Limit afternoon naps.

Plan activities like bathing, exercise, and visits for early in the day.

Set peaceful evening mood, keep lights low, reduce noise, play soothing music.

Limit caffeine.

Alleviate pain.

Maintain a comfortable bedroom temperature.

Use nightlights in bedrooms, hall, and bathrooms.

Ask your doctor for advice.

Bathroom and Beyond

As a couple progresses in their intimacy and years together, bathroom activities seem to get less and less private. That version of reality is absolutely annihilated when one of the people can no longer move their body. It is very difficult to become your partner's active extremities in regular life, let alone in the sacred private world of the bathroom. Nevertheless, you throw most of your fears and shyness right out the window as soon as there are basic requirements.

The level of intimacy was extremely high already with Cindy and me; however, this part of our relationship put us in a whole other galaxy! Fortunately, as in pregnancy and MS, the progression is not too rapid, and you are able to adapt to the changes as they occur. For instance, at first I would just help her sit on the toilet and then help her get up. As she lost the movement of her last arm, I was called in to do the wiping. Remember now that even though I was intimately familiar with her nether regions in the lovemaking arena, I had never wiped a woman after she peed or pooped (I am a guy after all). The first important lesson was "front to back" and never "back to front" to keep the poop area from infecting the pee area.

Indoor plumbing versus outdoor plumbing (women versus men) is definitely an advantage for men—not to mention the urinary tract infections and menstruation of course (although women have us beat by a mile with their ability to breastfeed, the ultimate providers and nurturers)!

It was hard getting used to being the maintenance guy down there and then turning around and being the lover; however, the rewards were overpowering as usual for the latter. The hard part was having to help her in public bathrooms (ladies' room only of course), where I had to hear other women pee and poop. It's harder when they are not your intimate life partners and you inevitably have to encounter them face-to-face on the way out of the stall!

The fact that Cindy's ability to help herself progressively diminished over time made it easier for me to get used to all the stages of assistance that I would ultimately have to provide. As she really lost control with time (and fought feverishly to avoid catheters), I was called on to actually push on her stomach with my hands with all my strength and weight to evacuate both pee and poop to make sure she was functioning and remained relatively healthy. This was extremely hard at first as you might imagine; however, keeping her healthy and off catheters was our reward. Also, our house is situated with a powerful trade wind flowing right out the bathroom window, so the olfactory issues were minimized (plus, as we all know, our partner's shit doesn't smell anyway)!

Just as in the deepest and darkest part of child-rearing, when the baby is going off for the tenth time in the middle of the night, we found it best to just laugh at the situation. It was comical in how absurd the whole thing was; however, it was very beautiful for me to be able to step up and provide her with the movement she no longer possessed. We were a true team on every level, and the level of intimacy was indescribable.

There were other parts of the bathroom activity that were much easier, like putting Cindy's makeup on before we went out on the town. Once again, as a guy, like most guys, I had never put makeup on. I had to learn all about rouge, base, mascara, lipstick, and all other beauty secrets. I also became pretty good at eyebrow plucking and hairstyling, including the art of using scrunchies and hair clips. That was the easy part, as I enjoyed the creative part of dressing Cindy up to the nines, including the mastering of putting a bra on (I was fairly adept at taking them off; however, I never had put them on a woman before). The fruits of my labor paid off when we would go out and she looked fantastic.

We would occasionally end up at nightclub-type setting where everyone would be dancing and trying to hook up. Cindy once asked me why didn't we just cut to the chase and make out, since that was what everyone was looking to achieve in the bar and club setting. We had fun smooching it up, especially since at that point, with her seated out of her wheelchair and in a booth, no one could tell that she had so many physical challenges. Her mouth and lips worked perfectly throughout. This technique was also utilized effectively in her convertible, as once I got her in the car with the top down and her wheelchair in the trunk, she was just a smoking-hot babe with her hair blowing in the wind as we drove to the North Shore.

Public Bathrooms

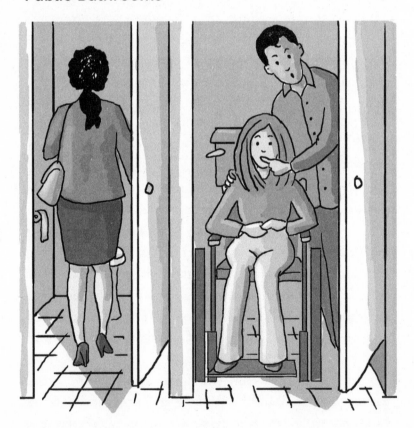

Once in the stall, the strategy consisted of me not talking at all—I didn't like to freak out the women in the stall next to us. I transferred Cindy from the wheelchair to the toilet, being careful not to let anything hit the floor of course, with Cindy constantly providing detailed instruction. The problem was that I couldn't respond to her questions without speaking.

As I pointed out to Cindy, a woman's lower anatomy is like a temple to guys, and we don't necessarily want to mix those applications up. In the early days, it was hard being there on the front lines with Cindy, but I got used to it; however, it is much more awkward to hear strangers and knowing that if you don't time your exit from the stall, you may have a face-to-face encounter with the person in the stall next to you after they have done their thing.

Of course observing childbirth and changing diapers prepared me for some of this, but the potpie/poop encounter with a female stranger in a women's bathroom was pretty freaky. Therefore, I quietly listened and plotted our exit from the stall and took a reverse beeline out of there! Although this subject might make most people uncomfortable, I have a whole slew of public bathroom wheelchair stories that are quite bizarre and maybe not appropriate for public consumption.

Bathing

I love being wet, and I loved getting wet with Cindy. That is the approach I took to bathing from the outset. It made it fun and easy. Cindy's skin was so soft and beautiful and was even more luxurious with added fancy soaps and shampoo products. There is something so primal about bathing a person, and I was a veteran at it, as that was my thing with our kids—I gave them most of their baths. As a surfer with massive amounts of hours in the elements (ocean and sun), my skin was nothing like the silky smooth texture of our babies or Cindy. Also, bathing a person is so pure and elegant, with the end result being a perfectly clean body.

My biggest problem on the bathing front was how physically excited it got me to wash Cindy's entire body. Of course it was easiest to bathe her while I was naked, rather than having wet clothes, and therefore I was always in a heightened state. I think this empowered both of us as it brought us back to our physical connection and once again, when we were both naked in the shower, it was like she was totally healthy. Note that to make the process of bathing easy, I tore out the wall of our shower so we were able to get the wheelchair in there to transfer her to a shower chair (a chair with what looks like toilet seat mounted on it for ease of access). She could relax in the chair and I would use the detachable shower hose and drench her with warm water. It was very relaxing and soothing for both of us (most of the time).

One of the things we struggled with on all levels was her loss of movement and control physically. She compensated for this by her desire to control everything else with her commands. I believe this must happen to most paralyzed people as they try to compensate for loss of control by grabbing any control they can capture. I had my methods for washing her and she had her directives for washing her, and they didn't always jibe. I think most guys are result oriented and most women are more process oriented, so we would often disagree on how to achieve any given task (e.g., how much soap to put on the washcloth and what direction to rotate the washcloth). After many years of practice, we would find a comfortable compromise on bathing (and everything else).

To avoid bathing and grooming problems the National Institute on Aging, https://www.nia.nih.gov/health/bathing-dressing-and-grooming-alzheimers-caregiving-tips, recommends the following:

Never leave confused or frail person alone in the tub or shower.

Check water temperature first.

Use hand-held showerhead.

Use rubber bath mat and safety bars in the tub.

Use sturdy shower chair.

Get soap, washcloth, towels, and chair ready.

Watch for puddles.

Keep sharp objects out of reach.

Have the care recipient hold a washcloth.

Protect dignity and privacy by using a towel over lap or shoulders.

Be flexible.

Be gentle.

Set a regular bath time.

Explain what the next step will be.

Use sponge baths if necessary.

Check for rashes and sores.

Seat the care recipient while drying and dressing.

Use lotion or petroleum jelly.

Teeth: Demonstrate how to brush teeth and brush yours at the same time.

Personal Grooming: Help with makeup and shaving.

Transfers

One of the most basic things a caregiver of a physically compromised person can provide is the transfer from bed to wheelchair, wheelchair to chair, wheelchair to toilet, and so on. Once you get down this basic move, the rest of the physical part of caregiving is pretty straightforward.

Being an inventor, I of course had my own techniques, and once again, Cindy wanted to minimize the use of medical contraptions, like a Hoyer lift. I observed how some of the professional caregiving helpers we had would perform the transfer, and then I modified it to fit my style and body type. Ultimately, it became like slow dancing in that we would be hugging very closely and I utilized my legs and knees as the base for the transfer and to free up an arm to position the wheelchair, toilet seat, chair, bed, and so on.

My basic move was to get her to sitting position and hug her, interlocking my hands right above her butt. In one smooth motion, I would lift her to her feet, hug her, and lock my knees around her for stability, making our bodies like a tripod and enabling me to let one of my arms go free and keeping the other one still hugging her waist. Once I had that other arm free, I was able to position the wheelchair, seat, or other object (including the inflatable donut, slip guard, or other pillow she would sit on) in the optimum place for landing. Of course, if the person you are taking care of is much heavier than you are, you will have to resort to something like the Hoyer lift.

The hardest thing of all, believe it or not, was putting or taking blue jeans on or off her. Sweatpants or yoga pants were easy because they slipped up and down easily; however, tight jeans were another story. The few times her other caregivers dropped her, blue jeans were the common culprit. The problem was that she looked hot in blue jeans (and always did) and never wanted to give that up. I got good at it; however, I would always encourage her to save her blue jeans for me and not her other helpers. I would always mix in something playful in all these caregiving tasks to keep our humor and intimacy. My move for the pants removal was a light tap or slap on her butt when it was exposed. This always got a laugh because it was kind of out of place during the seriousness required to achieve a safe transfer, and it reminded us of our roots as an intimate couple.

MedlinePlus has excellent advice on moving a patient from a bed to a wheelchair: https://medlineplus.gov/ency/patientin-structions/000428.htm.

15 Medications and Marijuana

Of all the medicine Cindy ingested over the years, and believe me any of her doses in the later year would have killed a horse, it was marijuana that seemed to help her the most with the least side effects. In the early days, before the availability of commercial-grade marijuana edibles, we used to make brownies for her. I have to caution anyone at this point that the brownies could be dangerous to the uninitiated, as who doesn't like a fresh pan of hot brownies! I used to label them with a skull and crossbones when I put them in the freezer. That didn't work all the time. Once one of Cindy's religiously conservative caregivers gobbled some brownies unknowingly. She got about two miles away from the house in her car and had to immediately find a bathroom and didn't know what hit her. She/we laughed about it afterward; however, it is a very serious issue. The other risk about making brownies for Cindy was that you had to be aware of the fumes coming off the pan as you could inadvertently take a long, strange trip if the trade winds weren't blowing hard.

To ensure that this didn't happen again, one of Cindy's doctors prescribed synthetic marijuana pills (Marinol) that we were able to get at the regular pharmacy! According to Cindy, they were good, but not as good as her brownies. I encouraged Cindy to try smoking or vaporizing weed; however, she had trouble with her lungs and throat, making it difficult for her. This was too bad because I believe that ingesting it that way is easier to control and not as long lasting as the brownie journeys (not always the best thing when you need to ultimately go to sleep or just stop eating).

Avoid Problems with Pills

Many care recipients may be prescribed multiple powerful medications for sleeplessness, depression, pain, and so on, which can be a problem for caregivers and a big responsibility.

Suggestions from the National Institute on Aging for Alzheimer's patients, https://www.nia.nih.gov/health/topics /medicines-and-medication-management, include the following:

> Compile a worksheet listing all prescription medicines, over-the-counter medications, and dietary supplements and take with you when visiting doctors and pharmacists. Give the list to care providers.
> List allergies and side effects.
> Take medications as directed. Ask for a liquid version if necessary.
> Use a pillbox organizer.
> Have routine times for giving medication.
> Place medications in a locked drawer.
> Have emergency numbers easily accessible.
> See website at: https://www.nia.nih.gov/health/topics/ medicines-and-medication-management

Save money on medications by checking out the website https://www.nia.nih.gov/health/saving-money-medicines for links to assistance programs like:

> The State Pharmaceutical and Assistance Program (SPAP)
> Pharmaceutical Assistance Programs (PAP)
> Department of Veterans Affairs
> Partnership for Pharmaceutical Assistance
> Medicare Extra Help Program

Section 3

Reach Out for Help

The best advice I can give to anyone going through a rough patch is to never be afraid to ask for help.
— Demi Lovato, *Stay Strong*

One of the greatest barriers to connection is the cultural importance we place on "going it alone." Somehow we've come to equate success with not needing anyone. Many of us are willing to extend a helping hand, but we're very reluctant to reach out for help when we need it ourselves. It's as if we've divided the world into "those who offer help" and "those who need help." The truth is that we are both.
— Brené Brown, *The Gifts of Imperfection: Let Go of Who You Think You're Supposed to Be and Embrace Who You Are*

16 Seek Expert Help and Advice

Seek Financial Advice

A financial planner will help you understand which of your assets may need to be liquidated to pay for care, the order in which this should happen, and how long the assets are calculated to last in various situations. If it is determined that your loved one may eventually require assistance from Medicaid to pay for care, your planner could be invaluable in helping to implement strategies which assist in preserving assets and/or income. They may also be able to identify tax management strategies during Medicaid's asset "spend down" or liquidation process. The financial planner should help to make sure that beneficiary designations on all accounts are correct and up to date.

The National MS Society website offers a PDF on adapting financial planning for a life with multiple sclerosis: http://www.nationalmssociety.org/NationalMSSociety/media/MSNationalFiles/Brochures/brochure-Adapting-Financial-Planning-for-a-Life-with-MS.pdf.

The National Institute on Aging offers detailed advice

on resources for financial planning for those diagnosed with a serious illness: https://www.nia.nih.gov/health/legal-and-financial-planning-people-alzheimers.

Seek Legal Advice

An attorney can help to make sure that you and your care recipient have up-to-date legal documents: a will, power of attorney, health care proxy, and living will. An attorney can also advise as to when it may be appropriate to apply for Medicaid, and may even help with the process.

Consider how your caregiver role will impact your finances. Will you be missing work to attend doctors' appointments? Will you have out-of-pocket expenses associated with caring for your loved one? It's best to consider now how your family's personal finances may be affected, and to communicate now with your parents, parents-in-law, and so on to avoid potential future conflicts or surprises.

Public Benefits

Check public benefits you can tap into:

Services for Veterans

If your care recipient is a veteran in the United States, home health care coverage, financial support, nursing home care, and adult day care benefits may be available. Some Veterans Administration programs are free, while others require copayments, depending on the veteran's status, income, and other criteria.

Veterans and spouses might qualify for certain benefits and other government programs; social security, Medicare, Medicare Part D Extra Help Program, and Medicaid are also available to those over age sixty-five or under the federal poverty limit. See the website http://www.benefitscheckup.org as a resource.

Community Services

Services that may be available in your community include adult day care centers, home health aides, home-delivered meals, veterans care, respite care, hospice care, transportation services, and skilled nursing. Call your local senior center, county information and referral service, family services, or hospital social work unit for details and suggestions.

Advocacy groups for the disorder your care recipient is suffering from may also be able to recommend local services. Contact your local Area Agency on Aging for help with caring for older family members.

Organizations such as the Elks, Eagles, or Moose Lodges may offer some assistance if you or your care recipient are a longtime dues-paying member. This help may take the form of phone check-ins, home visits, or transportation.

Many communities offer free or low-cost transportation services for trips to and from medical appointments, day care, senior centers, and shopping malls. Check with Catholic Charities, who help all denominations, for possible regular visitors for your care recipient and transportation.

Places you can turn to include family members, your church or temple, caregiver support groups locally or online, a social worker or counselor, national caregiver organizations, and organizations specific to your care recipient's illness or disability.

Adult Day Care

Adult day care could be an option for your care recipient when you're working or when you need a break. It also can provide your care recipient with diversions, friends, and activities. Almost Family, an adult day care center provider in both the United States and Canada, summarizes the benefits of adult day care well: "Adult day care offers a win/win situation for everyone in the family—not only the client or member who attends the program, but also for the family member who has primary responsibility as caregiver. Adult day care provides a much-needed respite for the caregiver, affording a break from the physical demands and stress of providing round-the-clock care."

Adult day care centers can be run by a government entity, or through a local charity or house of worship. The centers are intended to provide a safe place to socialize and have a hot meal in a protected setting. These adult day care centers are ideal for seniors who cannot remain alone, but are not in need of a nursing home.

Your local Office for the Aging will probably be able to direct you to such a day care center, let you know if there is a charge for the facility, and what the eligibility requirements are. For help locating adult care centers ask your family doctor, local social services or health department mental health centers, and Yellow Pages listings under "adult day care," "aging services," "senior citizens' services," and similar categories.

The National Adult Day Services Association website, https://www.nadsa.org/, provides names, addresses, and contact information for adult day care centers throughout the country. The site also provides seven steps for choosing the right adult day care. A checklist is available to fill out before visiting centers and a post-visit questionnaire is included to help in the decision-making process.

The Eldercare Locator offers telephone referrals to adult day care centers. Call the Eldercare Locator at (800) 677-1116, Monday through Friday, 9:00 a.m. to 8:00 p.m. (EST), and see their website, https://eldercare.acl.gov/public/resources/factsheets/adult_day_care.aspx.

Fees are normally quite nominal and are just there to help the center cover its own costs for meals and operating costs, like utilities.

Eligibility requirements will depend on the capabilities of the staff at each individual facility. Some adult day care centers will only accept those who are continent because they will not have the supplies to change adult diapers. Other facilities may require a certain amount of mobility for those attending (i.e., they are able to get out of a wheelchair on their own or with minor assistance). Give the center as much information as possible up front regarding both the fees and the physical condition of the applicant. This way they can point you in the right direction.

Medicare In-Home Part-Time Nursing or Rehabilitative Care

Medicare Part A (Hospital Insurance) and/or Medicare Part B (Medical Insurance) cover eligible home health services.

See https://www.medicare.gov/coverage/home-health-services .html.

A home health care agency can coordinates the services your doctor orders. Find a Home Health Agency at https://www.medicare.gov/homehealthcompare/search.html.

Community Care Services

Local senior centers may offer services on a sliding fee scale, meaning that what you pay is based on your income and ability to pay. To locate your local senior center call (800) 677-1116.

Some health care services can be provided at home by trained professionals, such as physical or occupational therapists, social workers, or home health nurses. Check with your insurance or health service to see what kind of coverage is available. Hospice care can also be provided at home.

Meal programs. Your care recipient may be eligible to have hot meals delivered at home by a meals-on-wheels program.

Religious and other local organizations like Catholic Charities sometimes offer free lunches and companionship for the sick and elderly.

Hospice and Medicare

Look into hospice care, through Medicare. This can be fairly flexible and a great help to caregivers who are taking care of someone at home. Hospice care is intended for people with six months or less to live if the disease runs its normal course. However, if you live longer than six months, you can still get hospice care, as long as the hospice medical director or other hospice doctor recertifies that you're terminally ill.

See http://www.hospicenet.org/html/medicare.html.

Hospice care is given in benefit periods. You can get hospice care for two ninety-day periods followed by an unlimited number of sixty-day periods. At the start of each period, the hospice medical director or other hospice doctor must recertify that you're terminally ill, so you can continue to get hospice care. A benefit period starts the day you begin to get hospice care, and it ends when your ninety-day or sixty-day period ends.

If your health improves or your illness goes into remission and you no longer need hospice care, you can stop it. You always have the right to stop hospice care at any time for any reason. If you stop your hospice care, you'll get the type of Medicare coverage you had before you chose a hospice program (like treatment to cure the terminal illness). If you're eligible, you can go back to hospice care at any time.

Note: be very careful when you tell your family members that your care recipient is going to hospice, as the normal reaction to hospice is that death is imminent, whereas that is not necessarily true.

Family and Medical Leave Act

Under the Family and Medical Leave Act, most employers are required to provide up to twelve weeks of unpaid, job-protected leave for family members who need time off to care for a loved one.

Insurance

For help with insurance rules and regulations, contact your insurance company. Many insurance companies will assign a case manager to address concerns, clarify benefits, and suggest ways to obtain health-related services.

While Medicare does not cover adult day care centers, Medicaid will pay most or all of the costs in licensed adult day health care settings and Alzheimer's-focused centers for participants with very low income and few assets. Be sure to ask about financial assistance and possible grants.

Private medical insurance policies sometimes cover a portion of adult day care center costs when licensed medical professionals are involved in the care. Long-term care insurance may also pay for adult day services, depending on the policy. Additionally, dependent-care tax credits may be available to you as caregiver.

Free or Discounted Services for Seniors or Caregivers

See the excellent website https://www.agingcare.com.

1. Benefit Counseling

Your local Office for the Aging can provide benefit counseling regarding health insurance, food stamps, and other services.

2. Dental Care

To find a dentist in your state that accepts Medicaid, contact your state Department of Health. It is possible for low-income seniors to receive a free set of dentures. In addition to calling your Office for the Aging to see if they know of a source, also look into your State Dental Association for free or low-cost dental programs. While not free, if there is a local dental college in your area you could get a substantial discount on dental care.

3. Elderly Pharmaceutical Assistance Program (EPIC)

EPIC is the name of the State Pharmaceutical Assistance Program in New York. New York is one of the twenty-three states that have such a program.

A comprehensive list of programs for discount drugs is provided by the Partnership for Prescription Assistance.

4. Family Caregiver Support Programs

These programs are often offered through the government, agencies like the American Association of Retired Persons, and volunteer organizations. Either way, as a caregiver, you can be provided with respite care by volunteers, as well as counseling and support groups.

5. Free Cell Phones or Discounted Phone Service

Lifeline is a federal government program for qualifying low-income consumers. To qualify, seniors will likely have to be on some form of government assistance.

6. Free Phone for Hearing Impaired

A new service called CaptionCall provides free phones to those with medically recognized hearing loss. You can learn more at https://captioncall.com/about-captioncall/how-is-it-free.

7. Supplemental Nutritional Assistance Program (SNAP)

You can apply through your state Office for the Aging or Elder Affairs Department or directly through SNAP in your home state. This program is not just for the elderly. Anyone can apply to see if they qualify.

8. Other Free Food Services

Check with your local Office for the Aging to see what programs are available in your area. Also try http://www.feedingamerica .org.

9. Free Hearing Aids

Try your local Lions Club. Most chapters either operate or know of a local hearing aid bank that can match needy seniors with recycled hearing aids.

10. Free Legal Help

Some local law schools operate a senior law center for low-income seniors. They can help in drafting a simple will, certifying a power of attorney or health care proxy, or drafting a letter to creditors. Another place to look would be the Lions Club. Many of the members of the Lions are attorneys and local business leaders who may be able to help you find a pro bono attorney to handle simple matters.

11. Free Medical Alert System

The actual system is totally free, even the shipping. The monitoring service is normally around thirty dollars a month. Check LifeStation and Rescue Alert, which offer this type of service.

12. Free Walkers or Rollators

Discounted or free walkers can be found at thrift stores, such as Goodwill. Hospitals and nursing homes may periodically dispose of reliable, used equipment.

13. Home Energy Assistance Program (HEAP)

Through your local or state Office for the Aging, you can apply for assistance either in the form of weather upgrades to your residence, known as the Weatherization Assistance Program, or as direct cash assistance based upon your income level. HEAP is available to both homeowners and renters.

14. Ombudsman Services

The state ombudsman's office is there to address issues with the care of loved ones. They will investigate complaints on your behalf to insure that nursing home residents are being treated fairly.

15. Residential Repair Services

Many Offices of the Aging run a residential repair service where seniors can have minor work done to their home or rental at no labor cost. You will have to pay for supplies, but the labor is free from the volunteers.

I have not used the majority of the above services so cannot vouch for them, but any help you can get is a lot better than nothing, and I recommend trying for anything and everything that might make caregiving a bit easier.

17 Nurses and Helpers

Live-In Help at Care Recipient's Home

If your care recipient is reasonably able to take care of him- or herself and has a spare bedroom, it may work to employ someone to live in. If you offer accommodation and a small salary, you can advertise for a retired nurse or nursing assistant. Friends of mine did this, and it worked well, though they warned to be very careful you check all references and also to make unexpected visits to the house to make sure everything is going well.

The live-in situation can be combined with arranging meals-on-wheels, a weekly visit from a volunteer from a helpful organization like Catholic Charities, and transport (also Catholic Charities) to a weekly activity group or day care center.

Suggestions for Employing Live-In Help

Ask friends, neighbors, coworkers, or other caregivers you know for referrals.

Post an ad at your place of worship, the library, or at a nearby senior center, adult day center, or hospital.

Look into a job-placement program at a college that has a social work program.

Run an ad in the newspaper or Craigslist.

Considering Applicants

Write a job description to share with applicants, including the tasks required, the hours and days of the job, and personal preferences.

Decide how much you're prepared to pay. See the IRS publications *Hiring Household Employees* and *Independent Contractor (Self-Employed) or Employee?* for details. For seniors, the cost of elder companions/elder caregivers can be defrayed in whole or in part by health or other insurance, the Department of Health and Human Services, and various state and nonprofit organizations that are designed to help senior citizens live life as fully as they can. If you are offering accommodation, the amount you will have to pay in salary can be substantially reduced.

Interview

Conduct the initial interview by phone. Ask about work experience, hours of availability, special training with an illness such as that suffered by your loved one.

Ask job candidates to bring a résumé, as well as names and telephone numbers for at least two references.

If possible, make sure your loved one has the opportunity to meet anyone you would like to hire. Watch how they interact. Look for patience, tact, kindness, empathy, ability to handle stressful situations, and willingness to follow directions.

Describe to applicants your loved one's needs, health concerns, likes, and dislikes. Outline the duties you expect him or her to perform. Write down the person's name, address, telephone number, and social security number. Ask for proof of identity, ideally a social security card. If not available, ask to see a driver's license or other photo ID. Ask if he or she has ever been in trouble with the law.

Find out if he or she has any special training and ask about work history, including why he or she left his or her former job.

Ask about his or her expectations of this position and why the applicant is working in the home care field. Invite the applicant to ask questions.

Be clear about salary and benefits, such as vacation and other time off. Head off any misunderstandings by addressing these issues directly.

Checking References

Always call references. Ask about punctuality and reliability and responsibility. Find out whether there were any problems.

Consider paying for a criminal background check.

Consider hiring someone for a one-month trial period before you commit to hiring him or her permanently.

Once someone accepts your job offer, put your entire agreement in writing. Include information about the trial period, job duties, salary, pay schedule, time off, start date, and termination policy. Keep copies of this job contract signed by both of you.

Try to be at your loved one's house for the first few days. Drop by unannounced to check on how things are going. See http://www.care4hire.com for tips on employing a live-in caregiver or live-in companion.

Physical Help at Home

Getting Cindy physical help at home, to give me a break, was an ongoing challenge. I estimated over one hundred plus have come through our house as caregivers of one sort or another in the last fifteen years! You completely lose your privacy and sometimes security with the less-than-trustworthy employees. We didn't have much money at all, so we were always trying to hire people ourselves (as opposed to an agency), and we commonly paid the price for not performing enough due diligence on the hires. Of course, it is a very hard job physically and mentally, and we weren't paying too much, so we ended up with some pretty marginal characters at certain times. The other problem is that Cindy (or the kids) would get attached to a great caregiver and then the person would move on to another opportunity or just simply burn out. That was always disappointing, but we became familiar with the cycle.

Some of our best helpers lasted a few years and became almost part of the family, whereas others only lasted a few hours and were complete disasters. It was frustrating, but the bottom line was that I couldn't do the 24/7 by myself, and although the kids offered to help when they could, the tasks were beyond them, and we didn't want to burden them any more than what they were already dealing with given Cindy's situation.

Hiring Help

You can try agencies for hiring; however, we had better luck often with the newspaper or Craigslist. The key is really digging into prospective employees' backgrounds and references. You definitely want to personally talk to people they have assisted in the past. The other thing we found extremely useful was to give them a trial period where they could attempt a few transfers and meals to see if they could handle it. The biggest mistakes we made were hiring people just because we liked them without ever seeing them in action.

As part of my strategy, I let Cindy manage her own staff as much as possible. She was used to being the boss of many people during her professional career running social service agencies and I wanted her to feel some of that power and control given that she had lost so much of that in the rest of her life. This was maybe not the best decision, as she sometimes hired the wrong person or mismanaged them; however, I think the overall benefit of empowering her to run her own staff was very rewarding to her. The other thing we learned was that if someone is not working out, don't wait on moving on to the next person. We made that mistake a few times, where we felt indebted to a person who simply couldn't do the job well.

See the AARP website: https://www.aarp.org/caregiving/home-care/info-2018/hiring-caregiver.html.

Privacy

Privacy was one of our biggest losses and something we were forced to get used to on many levels. On the basic level, Cindy's privacy had to be surrendered for her helpers to assist her when I wasn't present. She got used to it, as she had no other choice. Over the years, we became more and more protective of what little privacy we had left, especially relative to social situations. Even in our house in the later years, Cindy moved from hanging out essentially on our lanai, where neighbors would pass and wave hello, to the upstairs bedroom/balcony where she didn't have to extend the simple neighborly pleasantries that she got tired of. It is difficult to always have to put on a positive or pleasant face to people you don't know that well, not to mention that absolute burnout point she got to with the looks of pity she would receive.

I never realized how private a person I was personally until years of having to greet her daily helpers or visitors became extremely tiring. Imagine having strangers in your house all the time. Even though they were there to help us, it was a drag. There was a lot of free time when Cindy would be taking a nap or just relaxing, and during those times the helpers would want to be social and I felt bad if I didn't engage. I enjoyed meeting the various types of people who came to our house, and I definitely appreciated their assistance; however, if I had to do it over again I would have been much less available in order to preserve my own privacy baseline.

Help from Family

I found it useful to explore what each family member could offer and avoid areas where they had no strength or comfort level. Drawing on the strength of your family unit is a key asset in any caregiving journey, regardless of whether it is the family unit you created with your partner or the ones that you respectively came from. It is important to recognize that not every family member, or person in general, is equipped to deal with a challenging situation like a devastating illness and/or paralysis.

First and foremost, family members are fantastic sounding boards when you just want to vent your frustrations, as they will always accept you and not judge you too harshly. In our case, my family was fantastic in their handling of the initial news of Cindy's illness and throughout the struggle. I could always rely on them to pick up the phone and listen to the latest updates and/or brainstorm with me on how I could handle whatever phase of the journey we were in at that moment. Cindy's family was equally supportive, and I found it useful to let them really step up for some of the emotional support.

I felt like my role with Cindy was that of the overall provider of course, but also a little like a drill sergeant. It was useful to encourage her to push ahead and not feel sorry for herself. I encouraged her to call on her family to provide some of the emotional support and even sympathy that I purposefully stayed away from as I tried to keep her tough, resilient, and always looking forward with the eyes on the big prize—raising our healthy family! Even when Cindy was first diagnosed, our big relief and rationalization was that at least it wasn't one of our children that had an illness! Along those same lines, we pushed all along to raise the kids from four and seven years old through to adulthood with the best possible chance of becoming well-adjusted dynamic adults with minimal emotional baggage from having grown up with a parent with a debilitating illness.

18 Doctors

I think at last count, Cindy had approximately fifty doctors and approximately two hundred helpers over the nineteen years of her MS journey. From the first doctor, who really lacked compassion and delivered a cold matter-of-fact diagnosis of "multiple sclerosis," to the most caring, fully engaged doctors at the end through hospice, we saw the full spectrum.

The good news is that there is no rule that says you can't switch doctors, and Cindy lived by that mantra. If a doctor pissed her off, she was out of there. The real problem was doctors versus healers, and as she got more desperate and as western medicine continued to fail her, she gravitated (not levitated) to people who were essentially selling her snake oil. It was so hard for me as a scientist to watch this process unfold; however, there was no way I was going to deny her the dream of chasing rainbows and a cure! I would typically voice my objection one or two times early and then just shut up. My eyes were on the long game, having her live as long and as good a life as possible while we navigated our kids from small children to adults. Forget the money or whether I was right about the assorted quacks that seemed to endlessly find her.

Ultimately, she traveled to the Middle East and visited quasi opium dens in Honolulu, all with limited results. It was difficult not to mistake feeling better (reducing pain or discomfort), which is great of course, with actually healing the disease—a huge difference! My mantra used to be, "If they could actually cure MS, they would be on the cover of *Time* magazine!" Regardless of "Quacks 'R' Us," it was very useful to keep rotating doctors in (and out) because it gave her an added sense of control and possibility.

In a long-term battle like this, your doctors also become part of your family or team, and therefore it is important that you are completely comfortable with them. In many cases, Cindy's doctors became good friends of ours and really worked tirelessly to help her, going way beyond the call of duty.

The same rules apply for the caregivers (aside from myself, as I was a fixture that was not easily rotated in or out). Some were better than others in performing the tasks with the transfers being the most critical. However, some of the caregivers provided incredible social benefit, mainly laughter or the ability for Cindy to mentor them as young adults. Those were the two most important nontechnical skills we both looked for. If I could hear Cindy and her helper laughing all day, that was music to my ears. Cindy had a gift as a counselor and she shared it with many of her helpers, especially the young, more impressionable ones. She was a great role model too as someone who really got the short end of the straw but kept her sense of humor and overall cutting social edge.

She was a "take-no-prisoners" woman and instilled that feminist power in many of the two-hundred-plus women who came through our doors. On the flip side, she was brutally tough to some of them and either gave them such a hard time they would come crying to me or they would just outright quit, if Cindy didn't fire them first. She was essentially running a care home for herself, funded and supported by me— the one built-in resident caregiver. I highly recommend letting the person being cared for have as much control over *anything* possible to sustain their feelings as a functioning human who is part of family.

The other thing Cindy controlled, against my primitive instincts, was her beauty procedures. She had the best hair dresser and eyebrow person on the island, and although it was costly it provided two huge benefits: she felt (and was) beautiful for the parts of her body that could be controlled, and of course that was a boon for me, as I never lost my primal, massive attraction to her (although I also liked her when her hair was wild and crazy)!

Dealing with Doctors

Dealing with doctors of all sorts from the initial diagnosis to the advancement of the disease was a real eye-opener. First of all, doctors definitely need some instruction on human feelings and caring. They could be so cold at times, and that was a real turnoff for Cindy, especially.

As the disease progressed and we had listened to and followed the instruction of doctors from all walks of life, it became very frustrating that they didn't seem to have anything to help her aside from the usual pharmaceuticals. At one point, Cindy actually abandoned western medicine completely and explored numerous alternative approaches. Most of the doctors (western and eastern) helped her live with her situation and the pain; however, none of them could prevent the inevitable decline of her condition. Cindy got the short straw when it came to MS, primary progressive, not the mild or relapsing and remitting versions. I think the type of MS Cindy had preordained her disappointment with her doctors, as they were never in a position to change the outcome, only help her live with it as it progressed. Once she accepted that fact, it was a lot easier to understand where the doctors were coming from.

Choosing a Doctor

Good health care requires a partnership between the patient, family, and physician. You want a doctor who is competent and well trained in the types of health issues you have. You also want one who gives you the time necessary to listen to and address your health problems or questions.

If you have a family doctor that you know and trust, you may want to ask him or her for a referral to a doctor who specializes in your care recipient's illness. You could also ask friends for recommendations. Your doctor must be someone you can trust and rely on. If you are dissatisfied with the level of treatment you are getting, then by all means seek out a new doctor and a second, and even third, opinion.

Call the doctor's office to speak with an office manager who can provide details about the doctor's credentials, office policies, and payment procedures. Check to see what board certifications the doctor has. It is important, too, to be satisfied with the doctor's staff, as you will also be dealing with them.

Talk to your doctor or doctor's staff and your insurance company about what is covered and what tests, for instance diagnostic tests, are covered.

Medicare, the government's health insurance program for people sixty-five and up, and Medicaid, the joint federal-state medical-assistance program for people with limited income or assets, typically reimburse doctors for a diagnostic assessment and certain medical tests needed to determine if a patient has Alzheimer's disease, provided your doctor accepts these plans as payment. Again, talk to your doctor or doctor's staff about what is covered.

Doctor's Visits

When visiting doctors, write down what you'd like to discuss and bring the list to your appointment.

Prepare a list of concerns.

Make sure you understand all treatment options, as well as the risks and benefits of each.

Bring a list of medications. including dosages, with you to each appointment.

After each appointment, make sure to update your records with any test results or changes to medications or care plans.

See the National Institute on Aging website for further good advice: https://www.nia.nih.gov/health/doctor-patient-communication/talking-with-your-doctor.

19 Fight for Your Rights and Causes

One thing that happens to you when you are caring for a disabled person is that by default you become a type of activist for those with challenges. We were always willing to adapt to any condition we were placed in; however, we were always quick to point out to people or organizations that they should really consider making accommodation for people in wheelchairs. The Americans with Disabilities Act has made this situation much better; however, there are still conditions most people do not recognize. Our modus operandi was just to persevere and effectively make our point without complaining, but rather show people what it is like without assistance or consideration.

We were famous for climbing stairs in the wheelchair or carrying Cindy in my arms into establishments with no formal access. The owners usually got the powerful message right away. Our cause was to show that people in wheelchairs still want to do all the great things in the world that everyone else can do, even though people and places aren't necessarily set up for that. Our pet peeve was that people automatically prejudge a person who is confined to a wheelchair, and we enjoyed expanding people's perceptions on what wheelchair-bound people could actually achieve. We were well known for scaling physical entrances and obstacles, engaging in lively debates, and of course making out in public! Cindy was a fully functioning powerhouse of a woman, except of course for her arms and legs, and we were proud to show off her capabilities!

Section 4

Grieve and Then Create New Dreams

Caregiving often calls us to lean into love we didn't know possible.

—Tia Walker, *The Inspired Caregiver*

20 Love, Loss, and Lessons Learned

Nineteen years after her diagnosis, Cindy passed away peacefully in her sleep next to me in our bed on the day of our thirty-first wedding anniversary. The illness had run its course, and Cindy toughed it out until our kids reached the advanced ages of twenty-three and twenty-six—a long way from four and seven years old when she was first diagnosed.

We had been preparing them for years for that day, and they handled it well. I repeatedly told them in the last few years that their mother was dying and they should spend as much time as they could with her and clear up any issues that they may have had with her. It was sad, and no matter how much we prepared for it, it was and is still tough.

During the initial shock of the first few days and weeks, you seem to operate on adrenaline as you grieve with family and friends. It is like you have hundreds of mini grieving sessions as more people approach you or learn about her passing. There is and will always be a hole in our hearts. It seems to fluctuate in size depending on the day or situation.

We had a beautiful life together and we lived it to the

fullest—no matter what condition we were in—and we have the product of our deep love affair forging ahead in our children. All of our dreams and visions can now be passed on to them as the circle of life continues.

The lessons I have learned from this journey are indescribable, and even though I would not wish it on anyone, it was an amazing, eye-opening experience that has absolutely changed me to the core.

21 Caregiving, A Daughter's Perspective, by Kera Yonover

Caregiving has always been a part of my life, whether I was on the giving end, the receiving end, or witnessing it firsthand. My mom got sick when I was very young. Her illness was the type that is quick to progress. I found myself going from a care receiver to a caregiver at a very young age.

As women, we naturally take on the role of being a caregiver. Knowing this now, at twenty-three years old, makes me see much more clearly how much my mother struggled with giving up her role as a caregiver and taking on the role of a care receiver. My dad had to take on the role of a caregiver for not only my brother and me, but my mother as well—a burden not many would be willing to carry. The care we all collectively had to give was so much more than just physical. Every day was an emotional and mental struggle. Watching someone you love get sicker and sicker is one of the hardest things I've ever had to do.

In all the darkness though, there was light at the end of the tunnel. If faced with the same situation, I can confidently say that most people in their right mind would have cut their losses and walked away. My dad stayed though. "Through sickness and in health" is a common vow that people take when getting married. My mom and dad are the epitome of this vow. They both stuck it out and not only stayed together, but continued to find ways to love each other through all the struggles and adversity.

To say that the care that my dad provided for my mom was hardcore is almost an understatement. He took care of her physical, emotional, and mental well-being, in addition to raising two kids in the process. My brother and I helped as much as we could, but my dad made sure to never put that burden on us and ensured we had as normal a life as possible.

It's easy to love someone when things are easy and everything is going well. My parents were lucky because they enjoyed many years together before the hard times kicked in. How you handle hard times says so much more about your character and your relationship than how you handle good times. They both made it until the very end, and if that isn't true love, I honestly don't know what is.

Although my mom's getting sick was the hardest thing I have ever had to watch and live through, it taught me so much. It showed me firsthand what true love looks like and that when you love someone, you stay by their side through all the trials and tribulations. My mother's illness showed me how strong I could be. I am who I am today because I had the best examples of strength, love, and devotion right in front of my face.

—Kera Yonover

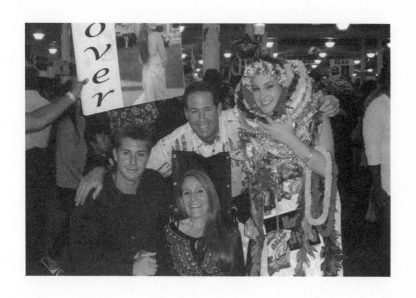

Index

A

accountant, 46. *See also* finances
acupuncture, 71–72, 74
adaptation, 48–57, 90, 131
adult day care, 106, 107, 108–109, 111
advice. *See also* help
    financial, 105–106
    legal, 106
advocacy groups, 107
airplanes, 56–57
Almost Family, 108
American Association of Retired Persons, 37, 113
anger, 19, 39
Ayivor, Israelmore, 81

B

bathing, 93–95, 127
bathroom, 15, 44, 48, 56, 89–93
bed transfers, 87–88, 96–97. *See also* wheelchair transfers
benefit counseling, 112
blame, 17–19
breaks, for caregiver mental health, 27, 31–37, 44, 46
Brown, Brené, 103

C

caregiver escapes, 32–34
caregiver health, 26–28, 28–29
caregiver mental health, 27, 31–37, 44, 46
caregiver self-care, 40
caregiver support, 35–37
caregiver support programs, 113
caregiver value, 40–41
care recipients
    counseling for, 39–40
    exercise for, 52–54
    favorite activity for, 54–56
    female, male caregivers with, 15
    mental health of, 63–64
Catholic Charities, 107, 110, 117
cats, 23
causes, 131–132
cell phones, 113
children. *See also* family
    as caregivers, 137–138
    frankness of, 36
    in home, 22–23
    mental health of, 62–63
    needs of, 25–26
community, 37
community care services, 110

community services, 107
counseling, 24–25, 39–41, 113. *See also* benefit counseling

D
daughter, as caregiver, 137–138
day care, adult, 106, 107, 108–109, 111
death, 135–136
dental care, 112
diet, 17, 18, 45–46, 85–86
distraction, 60, 61–62
divorce, 76–77
doctors, 28–29, 125–129
doctor's visits, 129
dogs, 23–24
drugs, 45, 100–101. *See also* medications

E
eating, 17, 18, 45–46, 85–86
Eldercare Locator, 37, 109
employment, of live-in help, 117–118
energy assistance, 114
enjoyment, 48–57
entertainment, 50–51
entertainment budget, 48
escapes, caregiver, 32–34
exercise, 27, 48, 52–54, 89

F
family. *See also* children
   caregiver stress and, 28
   children and, 25–26
   help from, 122–123
   keeping together, 76–77
   pets and, 23
   priorities and, 45
   self-care and, 50
   telling medical news to, 7–9

Family and Medical Leave Act, 110–111
Family Caregiver Alliance, 37
feeding, 85–86. *See also* diet
female patients, male caregivers with, 15
feminine side, 15
finances, 43–46, 48–49
financial advice, 105–106
food, 17, 18, 45–46, 85–86
food services, 113
food stamps, 113
foundations, of relationship, 3–5
friends
   in adult day care, 108
   as caregivers, 21
   caregiver stress and, 28, 33
   distraction and, 62
   losing, 76
   telling medical news to, 7–9
frustration, 39, 41, 43, 60, 75–78, 122

G
grooming, 93–95, 127. *See also* bathroom
gut check, 83–97

H
hearing aids, 114
hearing impairment, 113
help
   from family, 122–123
   financial, 105–106
   legal, 106, 114
   live-in, 117–123
   with public benefits, 106–115
hiring, of help, 120–121
Home Energy Assistance Program (HEAP), 114
home modifications, 22, 45

home repair services, 115
hospice, 107, 110–111, 125
humor, 10, 49, 63, 77–78, 91

I
"ignore and distract," 60, 61–62
income taxes, 46, 105, 112
instincts, 84
insurance, 111–112, 118, 128. *See also* Medicare
interview, for live-in help, 118–119
isolation, 37

J
joy niche, 49

L
legal advice, 106
legal help, 114
levity, 49. *See also* humor
Lifeline (federal program), 113
LifeStation, 114
live-in help, 117–123
long-term conditions, 9–11
loss, 75–78, 135–136
Lovato, Demi, 103

M
makeup, 91. *See also* bathroom; grooming
male caregivers, of female patients, 15
marijuana, 99–101
Medicaid, 105, 106–107, 111, 112, 129
medical alert system, 114
medical news
    dealing with, 7–11
    telling family and friends, 7–9
Medicare, 106–107, 109, 110–111, 129

medications, 86, 100–101, 129. *See also* drugs
mental health, 59–64
    breaks, for caregiver, 31–37
    of care recipient, 63–64
    of children, 62–63
    social aspect of, 65–68
    of team, 24–25
modifications, to home, 22, 45
movies, 32

N
National Adult Day Services, 108–109
nature, 27–28, 33–35
news. *See* medical news
Newton, John, 81
nursing, in-home, 43, 71, 109, 117–123
Nursing Home Without Walls, 44
nutrition, 17, 18, 45–46, 85–86

O
ombudsman services, 115
online support groups, 37, 107

P
parenting, 25–26, 33. *See also* children; family
patients. *See* care recipients
pets, 23–24
phone service, 113
pills, 100–101. *See also* drugs; medications
preparation, 21–29
priorities, in finances, 45–46
privacy, 14, 89, 95, 120, 121–122
public bathroom, 92–93. *See also* bathroom
public benefits, 106–115. *See also* Medicaid; Medicare

Q
quack medicine, 73–74, 125

R
references, for live-in help, 119
rehabilitative care, 109
repair services, home, 115
Rescue Alert, 114
resentment, 19
residential repair services, 115
rights, 131–132
rollators, 114

S
self-care, 40
shopping, 45–46, 50, 51
short-term conditions, 9–11
sleeping, 28, 86–89
social aspect, of mental health,
    65–68
spending, wise, 44–45. *See also*
    finances
state programs, 44–45
Supplemental Nutritional
    Assistance Program (SNAP),
    113
support groups, online, 37, 107

T
taking stock, 21–29
taxes, 46, 105, 112

team, mental health of, 24–25
toilet, 89–93. *See also* bathroom
transfers, 14, 56, 65, 87–88,
    96–97, 126
travel, 56–57

V
value, of caregiver contribution,
    40–41
veterans, 106–107
village, 35–37
visitors, 66–67

W
Walker, Tia, 133
walkers, 9, 13, 114
Wallace, David Foster, 1
Weatherization Assistance
    Program, 114
wheelchair transfers, 14, 56, 65,
    87, 96–97, 126
Winchell, Walter, 1

Y
Yonover, Kera, 137–138

Z
Zamperini, Louie, 67–68

Notes

Notes

Notes

Notes

Notes

Notes